The Wisdom of 33

compiled and edited by

Donald Francis DC

with

Hayley Dorrian
Naomi Mills DC
Mary Phillips DC
Clare Cullen DC

A CIP catalogue record for this book is available from the British Library.

ISBN: 978-1-8384188-2-3

Published by Donald Francis.

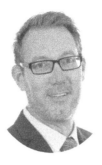

In loving memory of

Dr Dave Garrett Russell

"Chiropractic is so beautiful in its simplicity"

Contents

Introduction

Through the mechanism of the Chiropractic adjustment I, like you, have changed countless lives. I stay in my lane and deliver chiropractic repeatedly time after time and day after day and I love it and it has made me happy and successful in more ways than I could count. What I want for myself I want for everyone but so many young chiropractors are missing the boat and leaving without ever understanding the essence of our profession.

Chiropractic is beautiful in the simplicity of what we do but so powerful and yet we have for some reason decided to complicate it beyond fathomable understanding. For this reason, the profession and the world need the Scotland College of Chiropractic and many more like it. As I sat in the Edinburgh Lectures in 2019, I realised that I could not personally donate figures that were needed, although like many people around the world I do make a monthly contribution. As pearl after pearl of wisdom dropped into my brain from speakers I struck upon an idea: What if we could package years of wisdom from around the world into a book that we could sell?

We could bring the college into sharp focus globally, create something of enormous value and make some money for the college. As a coaching client and now friend of Ross McDonald DC over many years, his infectiousness for the project rubbed off on me and through this book I hope that it rubs off on you too. We have chosen to dedicate this book to the late Dr Dave Russell who was to be the first President of the College. Dave has left a hole that will never be filled but we will remember him as a person, a chiropractor, an intellect, a father, and a very fine human being. Bringing projects like this to fruition takes a team and I would like to thank and pay tribute to Hayley Dorrian, Naomi Mills DC, Clare Cullen DC and Mary Phillips DC whose energy and hard work has been key to producing this wonderful book you now read.

We have over 60 contributors from around the globe and from throughout our profession, some well-known and established, others less so but each has pearls of wisdom to pass on to help us all understand a little more clearly. Please enjoy this book and take something from every contribution, the ones you love and the ones that challenge you. Our book is minimally priced and if you feel the urge to be generous, then please do, in the knowledge that it will be used for the most amazing cause. If ever we see further, it is because we stand on the shoulders of giants.

Donald Francis DC

Foreword

Thank you very much for buying this wonderful book of wisdom. It has been graciously written by supporters of our project worldwide, as part of our goal of delivering a world-class, principled, vitalistic chiropractic college in Scotland. For over 15 years we have planned, fundraised, brainstormed, recruited, propositioned and more. The opening is now within reach. By buying this extraordinary collection of wisdom, from some of the most generous people within the world of Chiropractic, you are contributing directly to this project and, more importantly, to the future of Chiropractic in its true and natural form. Each chapter delivers pearl after pearl of wisdom and this will no doubt in time, become a classic in the chiropractic literature.

The foreword was to be written by my friend and colleague Dr Dave Russell, but sadly this book is written in dedication to him, his life and his commitment to our amazing profession. He has left an enormous hole that will take years to fill, and I miss him and his energy. As the person selected to be our first president, he worked tirelessly to help us over the many hurdles we have faced, in opening a world-class teaching and research organisation.

Finally, it is my enduring wish that you gain from the wisdom of these fantastic people, so many of whom have achieved so much for the benefit of the profession, and by extension, for humanity. Read it from cover to cover or one vignette at a time. One thing is for certain; your life will be richer and so will the profession, and beyond.

From now until next time, yours in Chiropractic

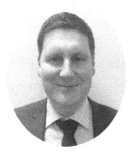

Ross McDonald DC,
Founder, Scotland College of Chiropractic

Dedication

This is the saddest and the proudest job of writing I have ever taken on. Saddest, because I have been asked to write this dedication in lieu of the foreword that Dr David Garrett Russell was scheduled to write for this publication; a schedule now and forever torn asunder by his own choice.

Proudest, because I now have the task of building a cairn of words to commemorate the life and contributions of the man who was known universally in the chiropractic world, it seems, as "Dave" and who I knew simply as my only son.

Dave, as acknowledged at his funeral in New Zealand, had serious chiropractic mana.

This is the Polynesian concept of life force energy and healing power, which earns its possessor respect and admiration. Dave earned this respect through a body of work which would be deemed outstanding in any profession: service on the staff, committees or boards of esteemed bodies of study in 4 countries; a prolific record of research with more than 30 peer-reviewed publications to his name; a mentor and friend to hundreds of students and conference attendees.

The 2 decades in which Dave made such an indelible mark on the profession he loved and lived for, began in the year 2000 when he became one of the early graduates of the New Zealand College of Chiropractic (NZCC). But he had found his vocation earlier than that.

In 1993, in his final year of high school, Dave was a long-distance runner with, as far as his coaches were concerned, only middling performance. He thought he could do better and set out to achieve it with, as part of his preparation for that year's cross-country championship, his first experience of chiropractic care.

The result was astounding, especially for those coaches, as they cheered Dave on to finish with a personal best time which played no small part in a class victory for his squad.

The flame was lit from that moment, a flame that burned with increasing brightness as he moved to Auckland for his studies, to Melbourne to commence work in chiropractic practice, then back to New Zealand where he soon returned to NZCC as that institute's Chiropractic Centre Director.

It was in Melbourne that another spark was lit in Dave's life, igniting the other great passion that defined his time on this planet; family and friends.

Melbourne was the place where Dave and Tanja Glucina chose to become husband and wife, extending the professional partnership they had already forged in chiropractic practice, to a parental partnership. It's a partnership which endures beyond his death, through the lives of their 3 children. Saskia, Oliver and Zara are the loved and living legacy of Dave's passion for his family. It is testimony to the strength of his many friendships that a network of mates and colleagues has formed in Auckland and beyond, dedicated to helping Tanja with their care, as they grow up in the shadow of having lost their father.

Dave made friends easily. He deftly built bridges between people whenever he moved around the world while on his mission to maintain the mantra he is widely credited with, that "Chiropractic is a f%#@ing big deal."

His loud and infectious laugh is a trademark fondly remembered by those who knew him whenever they gather in New Zealand, Australia, the United States, and in Europe. He was respected as a communicator and a catalyst in colleges, at conferences, in boardrooms and, yes, in bars, because the people he met there knew in their hearts that he respected them.

His devotion to the work which was so important to him, made him a constant traveller of the world, and he met so many people through that.

Beyond his career at the New Zealand College of Chiropractic, he was a board member of the Australian Spinal Research Foundation (ASRF), where he often served as a conduit to the Hamlin Trust, New Zealand's equivalent research fund. He played a key part in the development of relations between ASRF and the United Chiropractic Association in the United Kingdom.

He served with the United States based International Federation of Chiropractors and Organisations as a member of the Science Committee, and most recently as a contributor to an authoritative white paper on the role of Chiropractic in the Covid-19 crisis.

The culmination of all this communicating, researching and teaching would have been his appointment to the position of inaugural President of the Scotland College of Chiropractic. But this will never be.

We are left instead with the memory of the work he did for Edinburgh, from the time he became a founding member of the board of the Scotland College of Chiropractic Charitable Trust, through his contributions to curriculum development, to the hard yards he put in to steer the nascent college through two stages of General Chiropractic Council (GCC) clearance. It was all work that he loved with a passion and devoted himself to with formidable focus.

I gained an insight into just how formidable that focus was in September 2019. While travelling in Britain and Europe, I received a text message from him wondering where my partner and I would be on a particular date, as he was due to be in Edinburgh on that day. I replied that we were committed to be in Paris, but could arrange to meet him with a side trip on any adjacent day. "Not possible," was his reply. He would be there for less than 24 hours before boarding a flight back to New Zealand.

All that lust for life and work and love and family and friends and the future of the world came to an end just a couple of days before Dave's 45th birthday. Those candles were never lit, but the glow of the contributions Dave has left behind in the world of chiropractic teaching, study and research will never fade, while there are countless students and collaborators out there whose minds he touched. And his love will last in the hearts of his family and friends, the ones who can close their eyes and hear the booming echo of his laugh.

Garrett Russell
Brisbane, July 2020

Wisdom #1

Donald Francis BSc, DC, Cranio

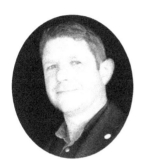

Donald Francis DC practices in the Scottish Borders. A former British Army Officer, he was born in Zimbabwe and qualified at Palmer College, Iowa in his mid-thirties. He lectures across Europe on many chiropractic subjects and teaches technique for SOTO Europe and for his own company, Veritas Curat.

Married to Katie, they and their three children run a sheep and cattle farm. Donald is a certified Craniopath and has a special interest in complex neurological cases. He is an enormous advocate for vitalistic chiropractic which is expressed through this book, his brainchild.

If it is to be, it's up to me.

Why are two chiropractors, educated at the same college, practicing in the same town, using the same technique, able to attract such wildly different numbers, quality of patients and abundance, therefore able to live such abundantly different lives? The simple answer is that it is because of "who" the practitioner is, rather than what and how they "do" it, that determines success. Who are you? Simply put, you are the product of your most common thoughts and beliefs.

While studying at Palmer College in Davenport, Iowa I was first exposed to the simple quote: *"It is who you are that determines how well what you do works and therefore what you have."* Or put more simply, *"Be, Do, Have."* At that point I did not understand this at all, and it was not until well after I graduated and had been in practice that it really came home to me how true and important this fact is. At chiropractic college you get very busy learning how to "do". To do chiropractic, to do one's technique, to become a certified bone fide chiropractor.

And then as I graduated, by definition I was a chiropractor like many thousands of others and I could "do" Chiropractic. But I had still not really understood what it took to be a great and successful one. To be great, I thought I needed more knowledge, so I did more courses and seminars in technique and adjusting, and I learnt to "do" Chiropractic as well or better than others. I also thought that success would come through hard work, so I worked long hours and tried hard, seeing relatively few patients, and becoming exhausted. I thought success must be about the words I used and what I said, so I practiced what and how to say things that I knew worked for others. Someone suggested that I employ systems to make my life easier and so I engaged systems that worked for others and they were really important, but still were not the make-or-break factor in me becoming more successful.

There is no doubt that becoming good and proficient in the art of chiropractic is important – it is certainly easier to be a great chiropractor if you are good at it. But strangely it is not an imperative. Hard work is vital too and it is indeed a quality I look for in all those who I employ, but again strangely it is not an imperative. Similarly, systems are a key factor that make a practice tick along like a well-oiled machine but in themselves they do not hold the key to the greatest success. What you say and how you say it is very important too, but again words, technique, systems and hard work are nothing without the intrinsic fact that they must represent your own thoughts. Therefore, if we are the sum of our most common thoughts then this is where we should focus; primarily on what and how we think. Our thoughts drive everything; our success, our happiness, the direction of our life and more. If this is true, then the most important factor to work on is... well it is "you".

And so, you begin to work on yourself but where do you start? Firstly, by hanging around and being near people who vibrate at a similar frequency to the one you want to vibrate at. Whoa there... vibrate at the same frequency? Okay, put simply, if you want to be a successful, busy chiropractor then go and "be" around other successful chiropractors, listen to them and try to understand how they think, what they think about and understand that in effect the very essence of their success stems from the core of their being. By all means mimic them, but only in as much as you need to, to move to a greater understanding of yourself and who you are and who you are becoming. After 3 long, hard and painful years as a chiropractor, I had attended endless technique seminars and was definitely becoming part of my technique tribe, many whom have subsequently become great friends.

My technique is very dear to me, for I have to an extent now mastered at least the fundamentals and it has become the way I "do" Chiropractic. But in the journey from graduation to that point, I had somehow lost my chiropractic spirit. My language was not chiropractic, my thoughts were competitive towards other chiropractors, physiotherapists and anyone who might take from the pool of potential patients who needed saving from their symptoms. I saw myself as the solution to their problems as I treated them and took responsibility for their ailments and pain.

It was at this point, as I attended the Edinburgh lectures in 2013, that I came across what is to become the Scotland College of Chiropractic for the first time. There I heard from people who spoke with passion and ownership of the chiropractic language and of the very essence of the spirit of Chiropractic. I said the word "subluxation" and I repeated it over and over again. I practiced the word "adjustment" and decided that both would be part of my lexicon.

I had become, in the words of Carl Jung, part of the "collective unconscious", as I had desperately separated myself from the uniqueness of Chiropractic in order to be accepted (which I never was) within the coveted orthodoxy of established medicine. But at that Edinburgh hotel I woke up and realised who and what I wanted to stand for and why. I moved miles in seconds as I realised that I wanted to stand up for Chiropractic, I wanted to be a chiropractor with no caveats, no apologies, with pride and purpose and understanding and belief. I decided that if I was to be a chiropractor, I couldn't be half a chiropractor and half a physio. I would no longer be what I thought society wanted me to be. I decided on that day that I would be something I believed they needed me to be, even if they didn't know it. I decided I would "be" a chiropractor.

I am reminded at this point of the fundamental truth as spoken by Victor Frankl the Viennese psychologist, who while being tortured at Auschwitz came up with the following: *"Everything can be taken from a man but one thing: the last of the human freedoms – to choose one's attitude in any given set of circumstances, to choose one's own way."*

I choose to think, to be, to act and to live as a chiropractor. From that day on, my practice soared and I have never looked back. I'm still not the finished article and I hope I never will be, but I am so proud, so emphatic, to the core of my being, to "be" a chiropractor, and I think every day about how I can and will be a great one. There are two ways to do everything, the easy way and the right way, and I have tried to make the attainment of excellence, the thots of abundance, my Chiropractic thinking, and the way I live my whole life into daily habits for if Aristotle is right, maybe just maybe, *"We are what we repeated do. Excellence, then, is not an act, but a habit."* Which then is the most important habit? Well, it must be the habit of thinking for that is who we are....

So, when two people within the same environment achieve such wildly different results in all aspects of life, think therefore that this must be because of something intrinsic within them and not merely the result of their actions. Thus, the evolution of my thoughts have made me who I "am", which has affected the results I achieve through what I "do" (Chiropractic), and brought me all the happiness and prosperity that I "have".

David Serio DC

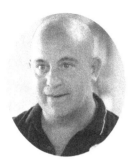

Dr David Serio is a 1999 graduate of Sherman College of Straight Chiropractic. He now practices in Buenos Aires and is the founder of Vida Chiropractic World Wide, a tribe of over 50 Chiropractors from over 18 cultures, currently practicing in Argentina, Brazil, Chile and Spain.

David is the author of "33" and is sought after as a mentor, coach, leader and speaker. He is the developer of both the Life Evolution seminar series, and the Life Evolution technique. He counts as his main mentors, Dr Reggie Gold, Dr Arno Burnier, Dr Thom Gelardi and Dr Joe Strauss.

Faith in 33 principles

Chiropractic is centred upon 33 scientific and philosophical life principles, which are the core architecture of our profession. If we are to have integrity as practitioners within this profession, these 33 principles should be infused in every aspect of our chiropractic practice. They are chiropractic's GPS, guiding us towards fulfilling our objective. The objective of liberating human beings from vertebral subluxations in order to enable the mental impulse to flow unhindered from brain to body and back.

Chiropractic is a human technology. The 33 principles are a human blueprint that reach far beyond the everyday practice of Chiropractic. They are scientific and philosophical principles that when examined and integrated into our lives, can serve as a beacon for our human endeavours and experience.

Here I will share 3 examples of how the 33 principles of Chiropractic can be used to reach a greater expression of health, personal growth and everyday decision making. My hope is that this gives the reader a taste of the depth of the 33 principles and inspires people to go deeper into these principles and their life application.

Let's start with our health. I want to give you a particular situation which comes about in almost everyone's life at least a few times. That is the experience of a fever. The typical response of most people when they or their children have a fever is that something negative has occurred and the fever must be lowered. I have encountered many people who have this point of view. I totally understand why they would see things this way if they were taught to see the body as a machine and a symptom as something that needs to be fixed.

This is where the 33 principles of Chiropractic shine. They arm us with a logical, precise and common-sense filter in which to see the body and its expressions. Principles 20 and 21 state that there is an inborn intelligence within the body, maintaining the body of a living thing in active organisation. Principle 23 states that the function of this intelligence is to adapt universal forces and matter for use in the body, so that all parts of the body will have coordinated action for mutual benefit. Once a person understands these principles, they can see that a fever, therefore, is an expression of the innate intelligence adapting and coordinating to universal forces. Therefore, it is highly possible that it's just a natural effect of the body's innate intelligence doing its work.

I have an 11-year-old daughter and the 3 times in her life she had a fever we didn't even measure her temperature because of our understanding of these principles. The first time she was teething and her body was changing. Her innate was doing exactly what it needed to do and on a scientific level the fever is a natural effect during teething, as the body cleans bacteria and other debris from the area. The second and third times she experienced a fever was when we ended long vacations and she had eaten a diet that was not as healthy as we normally eat. Her innate was doing some serious house cleaning as her body was ridding itself of waste and toxins that had accumulated.

Secondly, I would like to illustrate how the 33 principles can be examined and utilised in personal growth. I want to focus on principle 4 which is the triune of life. Principle 4 states that life is a trinity made up of 3 necessary factors, namely intelligence, force and matter.

Imagine a chiropractor wants to evolve in 2 particular ways: double their practice size and improve their technique. Principle 4, examined and filtered through the lens of personal growth, is a powerhouse of insight into what needs to take place to make these 2 goals happen.

Let's take each piece of the triune. Intelligence has as one of its characteristics, organisation. Where there is organisation there is intelligence and intelligence itself is the centre point for organisation. A chiropractor must be organised and have an intelligent plan in order to double their practice size. They must also study in an intelligent manner in order to learn and improve their technique.

Force: in order to double one's practice, we must put in force. Force will create motion. Without motion we cannot move forward. It's impossible. So, in order to double our practice size, we must find out what kind of force this takes. Once we understand the amount of force necessary, we must apply this force in an organised, intelligent manner to start manifesting the results we would like to see.

Just as in principle 4, force is the link between intelligence and matter. Without force there is no expression.

Matter: We cannot double our practice size or improve our technique if we don't bring our mind's creations into the material world. We need physical things to double our practice such as a bigger space, a better software system or books on technique. We also need physical bodies, we need people. A great question to ask ourselves is: which is the best physical matter to work with to reach our expression at the highest level? For example, which table will serve my needs at the highest level and which brings me the most value?

The third area in which the principles can be used to bring about a greater expression of life is in everyday decisions. I will use the example of a decision most of us make during our lifetime. That is of learning something new. Some people will choose to learn a new sport, or an instrument, a new language or to start a new business endeavour.

We find ourselves super-enthusiastic at first with our new endeavour. Then often our enthusiasm for the thing we were so inspired to learn, quickly fades. In studying mastery or learning something new, what typically frustrates people and becomes their reason for quitting, is time. People become impatient.

I have a friend named Robert who had wanted to open a restaurant all of his life. He studied and worked in restaurants. He was mentored in all aspects of restaurants. When he finally opened his own restaurant, he created this magnificent space that was his dream. Everything was going fabulously, except that he was going into his 3rd year and still hadn't broken even. The big problem was that no one told him how much time it would take to pass his break-even point and make money in New York City. He almost gave up. He was at breaking point, until he met a mentor who told him, "Robert in life all things take time. It just so happens that with the amount you invested in your restaurant, it takes about 6 years to even think about breaking even." This one piece of advice changed Robert's life and now 20 years later he has a highly successful restaurant.

Principle 6 in Chiropractic is the principle of time. It states, there is no process that does not require time. If Robert just understood the total truth about how much time it would take him to break even, it would have saved him so much unwarranted stress. He could have planned his finances better and made more intelligent decisions. This one piece of the missing puzzle set him back about 7 more years because without that knowledge, he made wrong decisions. He lost time because he didn't understand time with regards to his new business venture.

It is my hope that these simple examples have opened your heart, mind and spirit to wanting to dig into the 33 principles more profoundly. I hope you will feel how powerful a life guide they can be, if examined and applied to all of life's experiences and decisions. Albert Einstein said, "*I have deep faith that the principle of the universe will be beautiful and simple.*" That quote for me sums up the 33 principles in all their glory. They are beautiful and simple.

Wisdom #2

Billy DeMoss DC

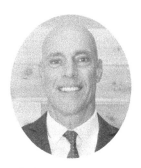

Dr Billy DeMoss DC has been living the principle and philosophy of Chiropractic for 3 decades with an exponentially growing global following. Either through DeMoss Chiropractic or through his 3-day festival of health, California Jam, Dr Billy is transforming lives and educating the world on the art and science of Chiropractic.

Billy speaks on many subjects, always with passion and purpose. He's an avid surfer, snowboarder and musician. He exemplifies living a loving, balanced, healthy and full life and is dedicated to helping people around the world find the same for themselves. Cal Jam is the largest chiropractic event on the planet.

Can Chiropractic and chiropractors really change the world?

My good friend and mentor of days gone by, Dr Reggie Gold, once said, "If you're not out to change the world, your whole life is literally a series of missed opportunities."

So why do I feel that chiropractors should be the ones to change the world? Because historically chiropractors have been mavericks, beginning with DD Palmer and his trials and tribulations in creating a new healing profession, being accused of practicing medicine without a license, and ultimately being jailed for it.

As Dr Fred Barge said, "Chiropractic can only achieve a significant role as an alternative healthcare system by working to dismantle the false medical dogma of the germ theory of disease, and providing alternative care to the therapeutic regimes of drugs and surgery. Our stand against immunisation, vaccination, fluoridation, excessive antibiotic usage and needless surgery certainly does not make us popular today, but soon the light of scientific investigation will prove the medical doctrine wrong. We, as the only significant dissenters to this defunct doctrine will be there to provide our unique healthcare paradigm. We have the alternative model to medicine's germ theory of disease, one that proclaims it is the "soil not the seed" that determines who will and will not get sick."

Chiropractors fought courageously to become licensed as a separate and distinct healing art, and generations which follow must continue this battle to ensure that Chiropractic is not diluted into the medical profession. The public is looking for natural ways of healing, and subluxation-based chiropractic is the solution.

Another huge mentor of mine, BJ Palmer, made a statement that really changed my life when he said, "*If the germ theory of disease was correct, there would be no one living to believe it*". This really conceptualised for me that healing is an inside job: "The power that made the body, heals the body." These were tenets that early chiropractors consistently espoused, an ADIO (above, down, inside, out) principle. It happens no other way.

Dr Barge also stated, "Healers lacking confidence in their own methods will have meagre practices." I know this all too well as early in my chiropractic career I lacked confidence and my practice was a direct reflection of that. I was trying to be the very person that our forefathers were fighting against, a medipractor.

It wasn't until I became exposed to chiropractic philosophy that I found my true self. What also helped me gain confidence was my friends and their mentorship. They saw in me that which I didn't see in myself; they saw my potential. They exposed me to different speakers who then became my mentors, and introduced me to the Green Books. I started believing in my abilities as a chiropractor and feeling comfortable that what I had to offer my people was worthy of their time and money. In the beginning, I was using machines and warming things because I thought time spent on each person equated to the value of the service I offered. Little did I know that I only needed my two hands, not electronics. In time my practice grew; the people of my practice started believing in me as they were referring their friends and families. I felt comfortable going out and doing public spinal screenings. And eventually I gained enough confidence to speak in front of the people of my practice by teaching chiropractic health education classes. Previously, the thought of public speaking had frightened me.

Taking a stand against the indoctrinated beliefs that Dr Barge spoke of, immunisation, vaccination, fluoridation, excessive antibiotic use and needless surgery, came with its own set of challenges that tested my conviction. I wasn't comfortable at first; what are people going to think of me, will they think I'm a quack, what if they leave my practice? A lot of insecurities ran through my head, to a point where I almost talked myself out of doing them. However, I made a massive effort to educate myself and read everything I could about the topics before I presented them. Some people weren't entirely convinced but most were on board and that's what I focused on; the people who saw the truth. The more I taught different subjects, the more people in my practice understood that health and healing comes from within and not outwith (the ADIO principle). I made sure they understood that first and foremost their nervous system needed to be clear of interference (subluxations).

My objective for the people in my practice is to reignite man the physical, with man the spiritual, by removing interference to the master system of the body which happens to be the nervous system. Subluxations are a dimmer switch to life, they keep people in a sympathetic, fight-or-flight dominant physiology which is good for short-term survival but not good for long-term health. As a chiropractor, my goal is to improve a person's overall expression of their innate potential by removing interference to this master controller of the body, raising their level of vibration and their expression of what they can be and their potential to not only be healthy but to have the most glorious, successful life possible. We are created to be healthy and to live a life of abundance; our body has the most amazing immune system. I teach my people to rely on themselves to be healthy not on outside-in mechanisms; to think again, always reminding them that healing happens from above, down, inside, out.

Teach and educate your people so that they can see and make educated decisions for themselves and their families. The people of our practices will become our soldiers, who will go out and recruit their family and friends. They will be living proof of these principles. To this day I continue to see my practice grow through our education efforts and most importantly through the lives that are changed. In my 36 years of practice I've seen miracle after miracle after miracle.

And this is how Chiropractic will change the world, by showing our patients how living a life congruent with Mother Nature will bring about health and healing. We can go out boldly and literally change the direction of this profession and planet by changing ourselves first and communicating exactly what Chiropractic is. It's as simple as that, it happens no other way.

Mary Phillips DC

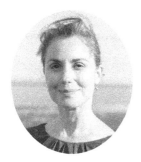

A 2nd generation AECC graduate, Mary is most certainly a well-being advocate, brought up with health food shops way before it was trendy. Acknowledging that we have the responsibility and power to change things we want, including our thoughts, Mary prefers to have a meaningful conversation than talk about the weather!

She has built two multidisciplinary clinics from scratch and now combines practice with coaching and creating bespoke meditations helping others to re-frame their views on the universe. Her hobbies include hill rolling, motorcycle riding and meditating.

Nothing is for certain

Have you ever had an "Aha!" moment? One moment, where suddenly your whole perspective changed?

My most recent one was admiring our fabulously lush, green lawn. I was so proud; to me it was perfect. That was until my then 9-year-old daughter piped up, "But Mummy what about all the dandelions?" They had been in my blind spot. I had been so focused on the grass that my brain had been ignoring all the yellow flower heads. Needless to say, the rest of the afternoon we were digging up dandelions!

This is a bit like my chiropractic journey. For such a long time I had missed the whole picture, but once we see something, it cannot be unseen.

As a 2nd generation chiropractor from a mechanistic background, philosophy was a dirty word. It was one I didn't take the time to look into, it was insignificant. My modus operandi was to find the pain, fix it and leave it alone. A "successful" chiropractor could cure something in just a few sessions (cure as in take the pain away). This view was reinforced when studying, as philosophy was such a minor component in the teaching at the British university I attended. I had disregarded it and it wasn't on my radar at all. It was just another hoop to jump through on my quest to get that certificate; to be able to call myself a chiropractor.

I didn't understand chiropractic philosophy, nor did I try to. A childhood friend, who went on to university to read philosophy, had a saying, "Nothing is for certain." How wise he was.

Once I donned that mortar board, just like the rest of my family, I joined a professional association that was mechanistic, with like-minded people. The talk at conferences was about how the other associations did things differently. They cut corners. Good chiropractors use ultrasound, tape, electronic massagers, cooling gel, and the adjustment is just another addition to those modalities. But I still felt like I didn't know enough. Good chiropractors have lots of qualifications. Perhaps if I had more qualifications, some more letters to put after my name, that would make me thrive? As I am a two-feet-in kind of person. I thought, bring it on! Every spare bit of money, and there wasn't much, was spent on becoming "enough".

Roll on another 6 months and if I'm honest I was struggling. I walked the 2 miles each way to the supermarket rather than spend money on fuel. I was not able to start paying back my student loan. I felt that I wasn't a good enough chiropractor. I compared myself to my peers. By this time, I had been on so many courses to better myself but the courses and the letters after my name changed nothing. I was disillusioned.

Insanity has been defined as doing the same thing over and over again but expecting different results. Hello? Time to change what I was doing.

I was offered a locum position for a few weeks, where I was guaranteed a match in my monthly income, by someone who believed in me more than I believed in myself. I ditched my associate position (where I mostly vacuumed the clinic, folded gowns and answered the phone when it rang) and I officially became a locum. I had worked in a mechanistic clinic with 20-30-minute appointments and suddenly went to 10-minute appointments in my first locum position. Ouch! That challenged my perspective, but I survived it. I had a constant supply of work, many offers of full-time positions, and had I wanted to stay working in the UK I would have taken one of them. I met some wonderful people and started to grow in confidence. I was on the road to figuring out what kind of chiropractor I wanted to be, what I wanted in a clinic, and more importantly what I didn't.

Still, something was missing.

A dear friend had a spare ticket to a different association's annual conference. It was a vitalistic one; what my family called "the dark side". We hadn't caught up for ages so I decided to join her, and that weekend was pivotal. The atmosphere there was phenomenal and the speakers came from all over the world. They spoke about a wide variety of topics such as techniques, communication skills, how Chiropractic actually came about and research too. It was there that I finally found out what it was I was searching for; philosophy. And with that came a belief in myself; that I am enough. Incredibly, it was by going to "the dark side" that I found the spark that has become my shining light ever since. It was full of accepting people who respected others' views.

I'm a breed that few people talk openly about. Maybe I'm a fraud, being asked to contribute here, Wisdom of 33. It took me an inordinate amount of time to commit to doing this. However here I am, and here you are. Spending your precious time reading these fabulous musings from some truly inspirational people. Thank you.

You see, I'm not a pure vitalistic chiropractor. I'm not a pure mechanist either. I'm about 80% vitalistic. I move along the spectrum, as do many. Maybe even you? It's just not discussed. I like the research but it doesn't always correlate with the findings I experience in clinic. Apparently, Chiropractic can't claim to help colic, even though I've seen these symptoms reduce significantly time and time again in my practice. How about that sweet spot when you've been seeing a client consistently for over 3 months and they realise that they haven't needed their asthma inhaler or perhaps haven't had a cold, the one they usually get every year. But according to current evidence, Chiropractic doesn't affect immunity. Houston, we have a problem...

I focus on my truths. I acknowledge the power that made the body, heals the body. We don't have to believe in Chiropractic, it is not a religion. I do acknowledge it works, and not just for pain relief. It's phenomenally deeper than that. I acknowledge that everyone is entitled to their own views. What are your truths? Your absolutes? I hear Dave Russell in my ear right now...

Everyone's chiropractic journey is different. Our clients' ones certainly won't match ours. One journey isn't superior to another's, whether practitioner or not. Within this profession it is so easy to focus on the things that make us different. Now is the time to narrow that gap, perhaps choosing to consciously focus on what brings us closer together.

So, in a world where nothing is certain, be yourself whoever you are at this moment in time. You never know what experiences are coming your way to shake up your reality and change you. Who you are now is not the person you were a decade ago and it sure isn't the person you'll be in another decade. And if you don't like the current version of yourself, you have the power to be proactive and adapt to become the greatest you.

As an eternal student I feel it is my duty to be the best I can be, for my loved ones and clients. Maya Angelou sums this up: *"Do the best you can until you know better. Then when you know better, do better."*

So, let's all keep doing our best.

Wisdom #3

Shawn Powers DC

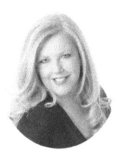 *Chiropractor of the Year twice, Dr Shawn is a former critical care nurse, marathoner, polo player and serial entrepreneur. A mum of 4 and a lover of animals at her home in California, Shawn is creator and CEO of multiple family practices as well as PowerSource Coaching.*

She has been a board member of multiple state organisations as well as the World Congress of Women Chiropractors, a Knight of the Royal Chiropractic Roundtable, the Leukemia Society Woman of the Year and co-founder of the League of Chiropractic Women. Shawn made history chairing the first chiropractic conference to exclusively feature all women speakers.

The "bigness" of Chiropractic

"He who influences the times in which he lives, has influenced all the times that come after." - Elbert Hubbard

She held her limp baby, tears streaming down her face and asked in a whisper, can you help? Her baby girl severely damaged at birth, suffering. The baby's life consisted of intense seizures, up to 42 a day, alternating with periods of lifelessness.

She had been told there was no hope for her baby, that nothing could be done, and to prepare for the worst. A mother, desperate to help her baby girl, coming to Chiropractic as a last resort.

There is no greater honour than to be trusted with the privilege of caring for children. As a chiropractor, it is an awe-inspiring experience to adjust and see life retuning, especially in an infant.

BJ Palmer, the developer of Chiropractic, wrote in the Big Idea: "*The adjustment of the subluxation to release pressure upon nerves, to restore mental impulse flow, to restore health, is big enough to rebuild the thoughts and actions of the world. This idea is the biggest I know of.*"

The bigness of Chiropractic is helping people who want the best for their families, and especially for those who have been told that there is no hope, there are no answers.

The results of this seizure-ridden baby receiving chiropractic care were miraculous. Since 1895, doctors, students, and patients of Chiropractic have experienced the amazing things a body can do when subluxations are corrected.

This has been one of the greatest privileges of my career, witnessing the joy these parents had holding their baby, seeing the ease in her tiny body without experiencing intense seizures alternating with lifelessness. Chiropractic care corrected subluxations so her body could better adapt, giving a child and her parents something they were told would never be possible.

The mother excitedly told the neurologist of the massive changes and improvements her baby was experiencing. This is the same doctor who told her there was nothing that could be done. She showed him how the baby was now at ease and rarely had more than 7 seizures a day and with decreasing violence.

She was astounded at his reaction. His recommendation was to stop care. In his opinion, Chiropractic was dangerous and not the reason for the improvements. In preparation for the visit to the neurologist I had prepared her for this possibility. She couldn't imagine, seeing changes in the baby, that he would be against her receiving care. His words fell on deaf ears; she was shocked at his recommendation.

In decades of practice and coaching, this is not a one-off incident. Unfortunately, myself, patients and clients, have all experienced other professions, relatives and partners who attempt to discourage, create doubt and instill fear about Chiropractic, because they do not understand.

It is vital to be able to master the ability to connect and communicate the purpose, value and need for chiropractic care and to understand the science that supports it.

To better serve mankind requires us to know and speak the truth. It is vital to help our world understand the value and relevancy of Chiropractic through honest, caring communication.

Science proves that Chiropractic affects our brain and nervous system, and due to this relationship, subluxation correction and prevention will impact an individual's health, longevity, immunity and most importantly the expression of our human potential.

The bigness of Chiropractic is powerful. There is no doubt that it increases quality of life. We have seen lives reconnected, saved, changed, and dis-ease prevented. As chiropractors, we have the opportunity to live a calling, contributing to mankind, and to live a life like no other. As a student or practice member, you too have the ability to influence, empower and support others with your knowledge.

It is not uncommon in Chiropractic to memorise quotes and have posters in our offices about the bigness of Chiropractic. We love them because we have experienced them, they are powerful and true.

After decades in practice, helping people experience health and helping vitality return, protecting and comforting people who all have limitations of matter, has been fun and rewarding.

Initially, I was a critical care nurse and once saw 12 people die in one day in ICU. It was heartbreaking and I wanted to do more to help people from getting to this point in their life. Because of my personal experience receiving chiropractic care, I knew there was a better way for me to impact humanity. I never regret leaving nursing, and would encourage anyone to consider a career in Chiropractic.

At the end of my brother's life when he was ill, disconnected and miserable, I was at his bed 24/7, checking and adjusting as necessary with the soul/sole purpose of facilitating reconnection. My family witnessed his dis-ease leave and his peaceful transition as he left this earthly plane. Chiropractic can help from pre-conception until we make our transition from this earth.

In Chiropractic we are privileged to care for a range of people: healthy people who stay healthy, sick people who get well, old people who become more vital, children on the spectrum, and non-verbal children who now speak and can be touched. These are not just quotes or slogans, it is real, the bigness of Chiropractic.

Success as a human being comes when we get to live and work with and for what is most important to us. Clarity for your personal mission, vision and life goals is vital.

Decades of helping others achieve success has shown that the strategies which consistently produce results are unmistakable. When we have a clear vision and purpose; the ability to control mindset and attitude; dedication to lifelong learning and upgrading skills; and harnessing focus to establish powerful habits consistent with our goals, success is inevitable. If you use these strategies you will definitely create an amazing life, vibrant health, and a successful practice.

Most importantly, as a person who helps others, it is imperative to nourish your own body, mind and spirit. Only schedule your priorities and know that it's empowering to get help and support to fulfill your purpose, vison and mission.

We have the power to speak the truth, use our 2 hands, our anchored mind and our loving heart to save and change lives, like the baby whose mother was told there was nothing that could be done. We have the power to influence and change the course of history, with the bigness of Chiropractic.

Hayley Dorrian

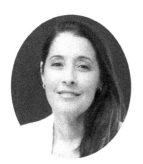

Following a car accident aged 15, Hayley experienced her first chiropractic adjustment and it has become an integral part of her life ever since. She and her husband co-own a vitalistic practice in London, while sharing two fantastic chiropractic kids, Hugo and Ava.

Hayley's passion and drive for making the Scotland college a reality, led to her appointment to the board of the SCCCT. She is also co-owner of the retreat and membership platform Hayley & Kelly which supports women and parents, helping them to connect, and explore alternative health choices for themselves and their families.

Chiropractic is not just a profession, but an expression of life

My journey into chiropractic began when I was 15 after I was hit by a car in a hit-and-run accident.

While the bruising on my body begun to heal after a few days in hospital, the headaches and pain in my neck and upper thoracics became more apparent. Having spent 3 days in a medical environment, I decided I wasn't going to follow the mainstream approach to getting better and looked for holistic alternatives. Among those I read about, I connected most with Chiropractic.

Some years later my chiropractic journey developed further when I met my now husband, Connell, who is an amazing chiropractor. Then I became a mum to two awesome kids, Hugo and Ava.

Having what I used to call a 'normal' up-bringing, my childhood included trips to the doctors when I was unwell, Calpol for temperatures and the belief that you need external sources to help fix or heal your body. But I intuitively knew that this belief system wasn't congruent with how I truly felt.

My real understanding of our body's innate intelligence has been tested and challenged on multiple occasions while being mum to Hugo and Ava. They are my greatest teachers as well as gifts to and from the world. But reading something in a book is very different to it playing out in real life isn't it? Especially when you haven't experienced that challenge before, and you find yourself in a system that expects you to follow whatever approach everyone else is, with intense judgment if you don't. The amount of times I was told that I was putting my kids at risk or that our parental decisions were based on incorrect scientific theories became not only tedious but soul destroying. I recognised more and more that my time and space needed to be filled with supporters rather than destroyers!

Although I knew that we wanted to raise our kids in a different way to the "normal" health approach, I just wasn't sure how and where to start, what research to do (this was before you had any social media platforms such as Facebook etc), where the like-minded people were and how I could connect with them. If I am truly honest, I often found myself paralysed with fear. Fear of judgment, fear of making the wrong health decisions for my family, fear of speaking my truth and the backlash that would come from those that weren't prepared to understand it. I found myself in a very toxic headspace and one that I knew I needed to change.

While Connell had graduated from AECC in 1998, a few years later he started attending various seminars in and around Europe. I noticed that he became more and more energised and passionate about the way he wanted to practice. He became more congruent with a vitalistic approach to checking, detecting and adjusting the vertebral subluxation. His approach in practice dramatically changed and he became a more authentic chiropractor and more connected to his patients, or as we call them "patrons". Although I was working on the business in the background, his energy became infectious and our parenting conversations started to change from, "We can't" to "What if?". Primarily it was my internal conversations that were changing; watching and observing the changes that were going on around me.

For several years, Connell continuously invited me to attend a number of these conferences with him, never insisting but always extending that invitation so that one day I might. I was very much sitting with the mindset that I shouldn't go. Chiropractic was his career and not mine and it was important to have these clear home and work life boundaries. In 2009, I attended my first UCA Spring conference with my dearest friend, Dr Kelly-Jane McLaughlin DC. I agreed to go, not to listen to the amazing line-up of international speakers but to help look after her newborn son, my godson. This day changed pretty much everything for me, regarding a real understanding of the chiropractic philosophy and why Connell would come home so energised after attending these conferences. Imagine me getting to listen to Cindy O'Mera and Sarah Farrant among others, at my first ever chiro conference. I most definitely had the biggest lightbulb moment!

So, fast forward and years later I am a fully-pledged chiro seminar junkie. I have had the pleasure of attending so many seminars over these past 11 years where I have been able to listen, learn, empower and grow. Not only for myself but for my kids, family and friends. I no longer fear being judged or separated from the pack for having different beliefs.

For me, another really fulfilling aspect of attending all these seminars is the opportunity to meet so many like-minded people. These are the people I craved connecting with when I first became a mum. The power of this connection among those who strive for the same health goals and beliefs have been instrumental in my own growth and personal development and I am deeply grateful for all their guidance, support and friendship. While some of these like-minded and amazing human beings are chiropractors, some are spouses or partners of chiropractors. This was a game changer for me.

I have often heard chiropractors share their stories on stage, in videos or in conversations about why patients come in for their adjustments but leave their spouses and kids at home. Why aren't they bringing in the whole family to get checked as well? This baffles some chiropractors. I share the same sentiments when it comes to spouses and partners attending conferences and seminars. I would love to see more spouses/partners attend these conferences so they can connect with others in a similar position, those with like-minded beliefs. I know it can be hard to find that connection outside of the profession and I truly believe that for chiropractic to grow, we should create a much bigger ripple effect, aligning beliefs for all family members within their homes.

Never once has Connell requested that we raise our kids in a way that hasn't supported both our own beliefs. If I didn't know or felt I wasn't able to decide on a health decision as a parent, I went out and researched it, I talked to people who may have shared a similar experience and then created various opportunities to make an informed decision. We did this together. I have had various conversations with spouses/partners about alternative parenting choices which they may have found challenging, having not always been exposed to all the facts or done the research. Chiropractors often have these learning opportunities working within practice or by reaching out to their chiropractic friends and colleagues. But who do spouses/partners reach out to if they don't have a like-minded connection?

If I hadn't attended the UCA conference 11 years ago, would I have had a limited outlook on health? I suspect that I may have listened to that negative chatter of self- doubt, fear and judgment and made some incongruent health and family decisions as a result.

I recognise that although I am incredibly lucky, luck doesn't come without focus and direction. I have invested my time, energy and money into listening, learning and connecting with so many lovely people within this profession. I have always tried to pay back the kindness that has been shown and expressed to me over the years, especially during the early years when I was a first-time mum. In recent years, Dr Kelly-Jane McLaughlin and I have seized the opportunity to collaborate on a project, producing a platform for people to connect with likeminded individuals and strive for better health choices. We recognised that more and more people are wanting to make informed health choices and not necessarily following the health patterns of the past. The best part for me has been building up those connections.

I have found myself being inspired by some great chiropractors. Chiropractors from around the globe, stepping up and pushing their way out of their comfort zones to share the chiropractic message on stage. I have nothing but respect for these chiros who truly want to make a difference in the world. I don't have enough fingers and toes to count the greats who have inspired me. A number of chiropractic female leaders have paved the way for me who I would like to thank; Liz Anderson-Peacock, Sarah Farrant, Jennifer Barham-Floreani, Alison Asher, Shawn Powers, KJ McLaughlin, Louise Sanders, Heidi Brown, Melissa Sandford, Mary Phillips, Charlie Moult and Naomi Mills to name but a few.

While I have expressed such gratitude to all these amazing women who have inspired me in some way, I also would like to pay tribute to Ross McDonald, Kevin Proudman, Tony Croke, Martin Harvey and the brilliant Dave Russell. Amazing individuals who work tirelessly to ensure the principles of Chiropractic carry forward for many years to come. Please don't underestimate the work involved in setting up the Scotland College of Chiropractic, it's a great deal of hard work, hours spent consolidating and bringing together all the requirements to work with different associations and institutions. It's painstaking at the best of times, but the vision and common goal will enable this college to become a reality. It has been an honour and a privilege to work on the board with fellow visionaries and implementers this past year and I thank them for all their kindness in supporting me in this role, particularly Dave. He was an incredible human being, a great advocate for the true principles of Chiropractic and will be sorely missed by so many. Thank you, Dave, for every bit of it, you were simply the best!

The commitment to, and investment in, this college is without doubt a higher level of kindness that is being passed forward. Not only by these great leaders but by all the donors and givers to the college. Connell and I have always embraced opportunities for ourselves and our kids. Whether they carry forward a career in Chiropractic or not, we want them to have the choice of attending a vitalistic college that supports and expresses their beliefs, should they wish to.

Receiving and paying back kindness is how momentum takes shape. I have to come to learn and appreciate that Chiropractic isn't just for chiropractors, it's for everyone. Chiropractic is not just a profession but an expression of life!

Wisdom #4

Sebastien Fuentes DC

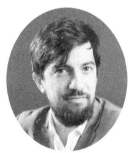

Sebastien Fuentes DC is a 2008 graduate of Institut Franco Européen de Chiropraxie (IFEC) and he now practices in Paris. His Chiropractic thinking came from "Life without Fear", other Green Books, the Chiro Europe community and from great mentors.

With his chiropractor wife Elodie he runs a programme called "Emergence" to help chiropractors in three principal areas: to achieve emotional breakthrough and healing, Chiropractic analysis and technique, and personal expression to fully emerge in their practices with no interference. He is a true exponent of living from above down inside out, something he hopes will make is son proud in years to come.

Light, love and life

"The mind, once stretched by a new idea, never returns to its original dimensions" - Ralph Waldo Emerson

Your soul, once stretched to your purpose, never becomes dormant again. Your spirit, once awakened to life, becomes unstoppable.

Chiropractic is better taught when shared through speakers and stories. It is how I learned it or rather how I started "getting" it. This is why this book will make such a difference. Once awakened to his true self, a man is free to achieve his dream and his vision.

Because, Chiropractic is not only a big idea (the intelligence). Once you get it, Chiropractic becomes a mission! It is the force that keeps you moving on. And it's about manifestation. You will bring your vision to life in order to realise your purpose, by taking the actions required. Because life expresses itself in matter.

Chiropractic helps people getting well physically, emotionally and mentally by freeing the spirit within. Chiropractic was born to reconnect man the physical and man the spiritual. The true gift of Chiropractic is not only to help the body heal from within but to awake the "fellow within". This is what sets a man free and gives him the strength to fulfil an amazing life.

Only free chiropractors can achieve this mission.

The universe and the "fellow within" talk to you in a strange manner sometimes. But get ready to listen to your inner voice, it can make a difference - I hope a big one - because we are here to serve and impact those around us, in order to elevate ourselves to a better consciousness through realisation, "bringing your vision to real world".

This is the story I have in common with my soulmate and partner, Elodie. I graduated from Paris' school in 2008 but I really started becoming a chiropractor a few months before, while learning to serve at the Panama Chiropractic Mission Trip, surrounded by James Sigafoose, Edwin Cordero and lot a great TORS. It's where I discovered that I was able to deliver adjustments and that innate intelligence was able to heal the people we were serving. I was blessed to adjust a lot of people. But I will always remember this kid, who was considered and diagnosed autistic, starting to play with other kids after being adjusted for 5 days. And there was this old grandfather with a cane, who needed help to walk to me and to sit on the table. What a joy to see him after his first adjustment running from the bench to get his son adjusted, and his grandson, because he instantaneously knew life had been turned on!

You will get that Chiropractic turns the light on, when you see the change in the eyes of those you just served. I really got it on another mission trip in India. Just go on mission trips! You will learn how to serve with no expectations, just the greater good.

Elodie is a second-generation chiropractor. She was already a chiropractor but she was awakened to her purpose in a transformation seminar built by her father and his friends. Being adjusted for a week in a paradisiacal place with specific techniques designed to awaken, saw her emerge with a deep mission: being a chiropractor.

Both of us are straight mixers; we are straight in our chiropractic philosophy and our life principles but we are so much more than bone movers. We keep on learning, digging, self-developing, to transform ourselves and be our best version. Our foundation is the chiropractic philosophy.

We understood quickly that Chiropractic was not only about learning how to move a bone, but that it is something greater and more profound that requires you to be the best version of yourself. So, in order to serve better and help the others heal, we need to heal ourselves first.

Maybe healing ourselves first is why we all came to Chiropractic? Once you get that, you start doing the work. For example, we have been to hundreds of seminars, and not only for the technique, but to be sure we will be very specific with every person we adjust.

We use a lot of chiropractic techniques from structural adjustment to tonal technique, and we've been to self-development (chiropractic) seminars, walking on fire, letting go of our old selves and moving on to who we want to become. We've trained with Demartini and Dispenza to go deeper into ourselves, to break through and manifest the life we want.

We always use things from the chiropractic eye to have tools based on the inside-out process because they respect the person's rhythm and the body/mind/soul/ spirit's flow. A technique is a tool, a modality. It's why and how you use it that is everything, and chiropractors understand it very well.

We started dating each other later on. Her father was already my boss and I was adjusting in the oldest chiropractic office of Paris, where legendary chiropractors have served, but that's another story.

In order to separate love from work, I decide to move to Barcelona and live my Spanish experience of Chiropractic. I needed to return to my father's country. After 5 years, we got stuck. I was running 2 offices (Paris and Barcelona) and we were seeing each other 3 days a week (I was flying back and forth every week). I was feeling tired, disconnected from my purpose, frustrated and even ungrateful. So, we decided to attend a seminar, a vital experience called Inner Winners with Marc Hudson, his wife Lynn, Chuck Ribley, Jay Handt. We wanted to clear our minds, to find our headspace and heart space cleared and connected, in order to choose the right next step.

We decided to leave a quiet and peaceful life in Barcelona around the beach and a beautiful chiropractic tribe, and get back to Paris. This move was not easy; letting go of an office built up over 5 years with a fantastic family clientele and a very good reputation was hard for me. We decided to come back to France not only to build our personal life but also to make a difference within the profession. We wanted France to become a strong and empowered chiropractic tribe.

The questions were: how can we serve the tribe? How can we impact to help everyone grow? Grow so we could be strong, united chiropractors.

Remember Elodie is a second-generation chiropractor and that we started serving at her father's office, the oldest chiropractic office in Paris (more than 60 years of service); it comes with stories and a legacy. And it's a peaceful place for Chiropractic and chiropractors. It has always been a place of sharing Chiropractic; we spent endless nights listening to wise chiropractors sharing their wisdom while visiting Paris, technique leaders, coaches, teachers. Many discussions and arguments over drinks with colleagues about what is the chiropractic service and what is a true service.

So, we decided to open our office to students and chiropractors for gathering and talking, inviting speakers to share their wisdom, their purpose, their service and their impact in the profession. We simply called them "les confs chiros" (chiro talks). We basically received students and chiropractors into our office after the last adjustments of the day.

What we couldn't imagine was that we were serving the community just where it was most needed; we created a tool for chiropractors and students to build their own vision.

That worked very well, more than what we expected! The message spread. After 6 months we were blessed to have Joe Dispenza as a guest speaker and lot of other famous people and teachers of the profession.

In less than a year, it became bigger than us; we received 500 students from a school of 800. We started broadcasting to other schools. But it wasn't about the numbers and the names, it was about the impact and the difference it made.

We share these numbers to inspire you; that a little thing with great intention can make a big difference. Listening to the chiropractic story and the chiropractic mission inspire, transform and awaken your vision, your mission. We can say that the domino effect has been amazing!

It made a difference and improved the course of the profession, at least for this generation in France. More speakers appeared and shared, seminars were packed and more seminars emerged. The result is that more chiropractors and students have been able to find their own art, be more inspired, find more support (between colleagues and students), be more successful and have a more fulfilled life.

The second gift of coming back to France was that we were invited to join a group in order to build the French tribe: Grandir En Conscience (Growing in Consciousness). We reunited and attracted lots of inspired chiropractors (those we met in the chiro talks) and students; lions hanging out with lions for a 3-day event. To that first event, 90 people showed up, the second 170, and by the 3rd, we were 300!

We have hosted more than 1,200 different people from the French chiropractic profession, when there are only 2000 of us (students and chiropractors) in France!

The service we provide seems to be efficient. People are inspired, they find their "why" through the principles. They are initiating self-care and self-healing on a personal level; they are building their tribe; they are taking actions to manifest their dream. The results are awesome: multiple offices are growing, people flourish and express their potential, chiropractors fulfil their lives!

"We never know how far reaching something we may think, do, or say today, will affect the lives of millions tomorrow." – BJ Palmer.

Remember: it's not easy to change the world on your own; you need a strong tribe. Chiropractors, once awakened to their "fellow within" and their purpose, are very empowered human beings. The power to unite a tribe can't be stopped by the fear of others. Share your truth and be surrounded by lions. Together we make a big difference.

I wish for this school to be the difference in our chiropractic world, in order to deliver strong and united chiropractors to make the difference within the world.

As with the chiropractic principles, The Destiny of Chiropractic is built upon the triunity:
1. Intelligence: a great vision
2. Force: chiropractors on mission
3. Matter: a united and unstoppable tribe taking all the actions required to change and heal the world.

We are a small tribe, but with great geniuses. We have a strong and constructive force to bring more consciousness and healing to this world. The uniqueness of Chiropractic is the most simple and replicable way to help human beings manifest who they truly are.

May this Scotland College of Chiropractic build a bigger and stronger profession so that we can all share the chiropractic gift: light, love and life.

Clare Cullen MSc,DC, Cranio

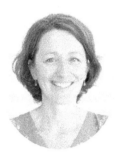

Clare Cullen DC is the owner of Ewell Chiropractic Health Centre in Surrey, UK. She graduated with MSc Chiropractic from Surrey University in 2004. She is a certified Craniopath and teaches SOT throughout Europe and is a board member for SOTO Europe. Happy to have helped Donald, Hayley, Naomi and Mary bringing this book to life!

Looking through a different lens

One of the things that has fascinated me during the Covid-19 worldwide lockdown is how wildly different people's perspectives are on the very same issue. Differing perspectives exist all the time between people, living at the same time, experiencing the same event. Influenced by your prior life experience, those most influential in your life, the place and time you happened to be born, your education and your ability to reflect and introspect. All of these will shape your perspective.

On my chiropractic path I have had the pleasure of learning from many great teachers, some who I have never met and many who I am honoured to share the pages of this book with. None of them will know just how much they have influenced and shaped my perspective. I learnt first-hand what influence we can have on people's lives when I left my first associate position after 10 years. During many farewells, patient after patient was thanking me for something I had said or done, and the affect that had had on their life; I had no idea! Never truer was BJ Palmer's quote: *"We never know how far reaching something we think, say or do today will affect the lives of millions tomorrow."*

I believe we hold a privileged position as chiropractors, to offer a different perspective to the mainstream story of health. This perspective is grounded in our philosophy and this is something we should hold tight. In the words of another chiropractic great, "We are the answer."

I often feel that I am not brave enough to speak out and publicly share my perspective on health. Especially now, against the loud prevailing narrative of Covid-19; that we are weak and must hide and lock ourselves away from the external invisible threat of disease. I do not share this perspective, instead I want to teach that we can trust in the innate, restorative powers of the human body. To share this perspective has in recent times been judged as unscientific or reckless, and even dangerous. I don't want to add my voice to the noise, or bicker and fight. I do not intend to argue or persuade people of my perspective but only to advocate for those, who like me, may be hearing it for the first time.

I distinctly recall the first time I heard chiropractic philosophy explained. It struck a chord in me like an awakening of knowledge or like remembering a truth that I had always known. To learn that a "vital" force exists within the physical material of the human body was not difficult for me to accept. One only has to witness death to see that "vital force" leave the physical body. To marvel at the miracle of conception and the development of a foetus is to know that there exists a mysterious power that works from the inside-out.

Within each of us who practises the art of chiropractic and others for who Chiropractic plays a vital role in their life and health, we have an innate trust in the power that made the body.

That trust has carried me through my life so far; birthing my children, nursing them through minor illness and even through the experience of witnessing a loved one dying. Ironically, this loved one experienced an awakening of this vital force that helped her to experience a deeper connection in her dying experience than she did in her life. The alignment of this unseen force and our physical body is necessary to enjoy optimal health. The deterioration of the physical body can occur in the absence of this vital force and we observe that as disease.

From my perspective, there does exist an unseen vital force beyond what we can see in the physical world. BJ Palmer called this innate intelligence; the organisational force in living things. Central to chiropractic philosophy is the principle that the innate intelligence of the body is self-regulating, self-healing and will adapt in order to maintain a homeostatic state of health.

We experience life through our nervous system; our afferent and efferent sensory, motor and autonomic nervous system. The nervous system is the avenue through which innate intelligence can self-regulate to maintain homeostasis. Expression of a vital life is experienced when the nervous system is in a state of ease. Interference to the nervous system's ability to self-regulate may eventually lead the body to a state of dis-ease and eventually even a physical body or a mind with disease. DD Palmer wrote: "Disease is the result of liberating too much energy, or the retarding - lessening - of innate stimulus. The former excites, the latter depresses vital force. The ordinary transformation of energy is health."

It takes courage to offer an opinion that is in opposition to mainstream thinking. I feel privileged to stand on the shoulders of the giants who had faith in their knowledge and the courage to share it with others. We don't need to bow to the mainstream narrative, which at the time of writing is resorting to controlling and censoring alternative viewpoints. To me this reveals a paradigm that is feeling the threat of the truth prevailing. Now is not the time to bow to a medical paradigm when its own pillars are crumbling. Proudly standing by our philosophy is more important than ever. If the existing UK chiropractic colleges are hell-bent on discarding our chiropractic philosophy, teaching it to students only from a historical perspective, then we are doomed to become extinct. Principled colleges like the Scottish Chiropractic College are essential if we are going to graduate chiropractors and not medicopractors or chirophysios. What are we, without our philosophy? Philosophy gives meaning to what we do. I believe that our philosophy is what sets us apart from any other manual therapist.

Another teacher along the way told me to "master your practice but don't hold too dear to your theory". This was a difficult one to hear, as the right brain in me is a ferocious reader and loves the theory. To offer my adjusting skill to help someone without any attachment to the outcome is one of the most difficult things for me to master, though this is in fact one of the most honest ways to practice. We don't know for sure what happens when we put our hands on someone and adjust them, offering an input to their nervous system. It makes sense to me that the adjustment will influence the energy of their nervous system. Their body will do with it what it will and yes, this can change the expression of their health. But can we always predict what that change will be? No. So, if we distil what we do in chiropractic to the "treatment" of conditions we do a great disservice to our profession and to the people we adjust. Any time I put my hands on someone I do it with intent and with love. With the intention of bringing their nervous system into a state of ease, for however long that eased state lasts, for that individual. Even if we can't say 100% for sure why it works, in Chiropractic we have a long history of large and small miraculous changes in people's lives - expect miracles!

Read and educate yourself. If you don't, then someone else will be telling you what to think. A trait I see in so many of my chiropractic colleagues is a deep love of learning. I have always had an unquenchable thirst for knowledge. At times it has been exhausting and overwhelming to always want to learn more and understand everything. I would often berate myself for my endless reading, buying books, attending seminars and gaining qualifications. I now accept my love of knowledge as a worthy pursuit. One caveat to that, which I have learnt more recently from teachers who have mentored me during the development of my new practice, is that dreams without action remain just dreams. So, while I love to read and learn for the love of it, I recognise that in order for me to grow I need to action at least some of the things that I learn.

One of the most obvious bits of wisdom I can offer is: get adjusted! I know I am preaching to the choir here, but for years I enjoyed knowing the theory of Chiropractic and had been in practice for many years yet still was only getting adjusted when I felt a niggle or symptom of sorts, which was in fact quite infrequent and so I was always amazed at how quickly that symptom went away after an adjustment. Since getting adjusted regularly I have a greater sense of connection to my body-mind-spirit in the way that Chiropractic was originally offered; as a way to connect (wo)man the physical to (wo)man the spiritual. The experience of getting adjusted regularly has changed my perspective on what Chiropractic has to offer and has been the reason I feel we must promote the teaching of chiropractic philosophy.

This is my perspective on what Chiropractic can offer; it isn't my desire to convince you that my perspective is right. I just need to know what I am here to offer and the people for whom this rings true will resonate. There is no "I am right, you are wrong", just differing perspectives.

Wisdom #5

Alison Asher DC

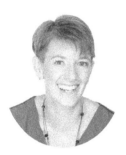 *Alison has more than 20 years' experience as a chiropractor in Australia. She opened an office straight from university, which she later sold. Alison worked as a locum all over Australia, until she settled on the Sunshine Coast working as an associate in a large office. In 2009 she moved to a home-based practice to be with her children and to coach with Quest Chiropractic Coaching.*

Today, she juggles the practice, two children, two dogs and a cat (and a very understanding husband) as well as Chicks who Click, a seminar and membership group focused on helping women click into the life of their dreams.

Big Bill and the first Chiropractic adjustment

What is Chiropractic? was written boldly on the whiteboard as we entered our philosophy lecture. We were intrigued; we knew what chiropractic did, what it looked like, but what WAS it? None of us knew.

"The reconnection of man the physical, with man the spiritual." - DD Palmer

Crickets

When I first heard this definition, I couldn't have been more concerned. I was already well and truly entrenched in chiropractic college and this quasi-religious statement worried my 22-year-old heart and mind. I worried that I had unwittingly entered some kind of cult, rather than a profession. When I thought about it, most of the chiropractors I'd come across were particularly clean-cut and healthy looking. A far cry from the GP I'd had as a kid, who puffed and panted when he wrote his scripts, and had nicotine stains in his beard. Perhaps I was in some kind of healthy sect.

Very often in life the things that perturb are the ones which grab your attention in such a way that they make you sit up and take notice. And so it was for me, for the next 4 years. That statement kept me awake at night and woke me up early in the morning, and started many discussions with friends and family. Was that really the role of a profession? How could that be? And if it was, what would that look like? What did mean to me?

Then finally, I was let loose on the public.

Big Bill was a taxi driver and he came to see me at our university practice for "slightly tight muscles" (he was bent over like a pocket-knife) in his lower back that were giving him "a bit of stick" (he winced at every small movement). He was sure that it was muscular (and almost every other spinal structure) but massage didn't seem to be working so he thought "a bit of a crack" might help. Before we started, I ran through all the tests required to make a case for care, with my supervisor. It was then I had to break it to Bill that we required X-rays before we could proceed. Suffice to say, Bill was dubious, and more than a little resistant. You see, Big Bill had been to a chiro before, so he knew exactly where I needed to "crack" him. He could point to the precise spot.

Big Bill was my very first client, and he knew it all. Fortunately, I also knew it all, so we were a great pair. First it was him telling me where to crack, followed by me telling him why I wouldn't be doing that yet, if ever, and that once I was cleared to adjust him, I would be checking his entire spine, whether he thought he needed it or not. Round and round we went, me telling, him telling me, and neither one of us hearing the other.

It was like I was at the top of the stairs ranting about how the spine is an organ, and that subjective findings aren't always reliable (so I didn't care about his symptoms) and what wonderful optimum function he could have if he just came up the stairs. I probably threw in a few unintelligible terms as well, just to ensure Bill ignored most of what I said. Meanwhile, Bill was stubbornly sitting on the bottom step, willing me to come down and listen to his story as to where his pain was, and what he wanted done about it, refusing to even look up to the top of the stairs, let alone climb a single one.

We grew increasingly frustrated with each other, and so, as the subconscious mind is wont to do, mine threw me an interesting one; that old buried chestnut from years ago. Chiropractic: *The reconnection of man the physical, with man the spiritual.*

In that moment, I had the first inkling of what the definition meant. Chiropractic is about connection and reconnection.

Big Bill was sitting down on the stairs all alone, without support, compassion or a shred of connection, and he didn't feel very big at all. He was fearful about his pain, his prognosis, his employment and probably even his mortality. On some primitive level, pain can stimulate basic fears, as we worry about being able to provide and protect ourselves and our dependents, or even being ostracised and disconnected from our herd. Despite his bravado, Bill was in that state of fear that we call sympathetic dominance, as well as being disconnected from his body due to his vertebral subluxations.

There was no way he could climb the stairs even if he could wade through all of that interference.

So, I went down the stairs. I sat with Bill on that cold and scary bottom step and carefully held his eyes and his heart and offered him ears that heard what he was really worried about. For as much as we like to say the concern is the back pain, or the headache, or the stomach ache, or the inability to do a proper poo, there's something hidden underneath the presenting complaint for every one of our people.

It's that issue that chiropractors connect with. The issue beneath the issue. The monster under the bed.

Once Bill and I were able to settle in and really see each other, I was able to offer him my hand. And he was able to accept it.

In that moment of acceptance, a contract was made between the two of us; the contract of consent. His rough hand held my enthusiastic one and although it's safe to say we were both a little afraid, we went up one step small together. Then another. Until we reached the point where we were both a little stretched. The magical place where there is both stress and eustress, and growth happens.

After all these years I like to call that contract: "Permission to heal, permission to help". It is where the person at the bottom of the stairs dares to look up, just for a moment, and imagine a life different and somehow more fulfilling, than the one they are currently living. It is where the person at the top of the stairs is humble enough to come down the stairs long enough to make an honest and truthful connection. Where they let philosophy somehow both lead and follow, as they see a potential and a beauty that the person at the bottom may not even be aware of, so that they hold a vision for the practice member that is greater than the one they hold for themselves.

It is where two humans choose vulnerability and truth, over fear and veiled intentions. It is a state of rapport where both heal*er* and heal*ing* come together for the greater good, and allow the innate intelligence that resides within every one of us to do the work. If it's done in flow and with impeccable intention and mastery, it's almost impossible to tell who is who.

So Big Bill and I chose to challenge and trust each other, and for two people who already knew it all, we went on an unexpected adventure. I got to perform my first adjustments on a "real person", and he got to yell, "I can't feel my legs" after I did them (oh how we laughed; well, at least one of us did!). When all the joking was done and the post-checks complete, Big Bill lay on his back and exhaled deeply. I watched as he changed before my eyes. Perhaps his pain was a little less, and perhaps he was content that he'd been "cracked", but there was something else. Something above that. Perhaps it was the bigness within.

Bill moved to that state of ease that chiropractors see over and over at the end of each and every visit, that which we never tire of. As the body is freed of encumbrances, the person becomes more of who they are, and to be the observer is humbling and curious and magical and grounding all at once.

Reconnecting man the physical, with man the spiritual; it's the biggest idea I know.

Naomi Mills MChiro, MSc APP (Paeds), DC

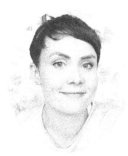

Naomi graduated from AECC University College in Bournemouth, UK in 2011. Over the next decade she grew 2 highly successful chiropractic practices while on a personal journey discovering the chiropractic principles. In 2020, she sold her home and practice to move to Edinburgh with her husband and daughter to realise their dream of being more connected to nature.

Naomi is an experienced entrepreneur, coach, speaker and writer and is currently working on her first published book alongside establishing her new practice. She also supports the SCCCT marketing and fundraising and sits on the Academic Board of the Scotland College.

Be Brave

If you are anything like me, graduating from chiropractic college didn't make me a chiropractor. Without real interactions allowing me to form my own opinions and give me much-needed experience, I was a sum of many different people's vision for Chiropractic. Some made sense, others didn't. Some of us go through our whole careers trying to emulate somebody else and never quite finding the fit. Others are simply paralysed by all the choice, all the noise.

Now, 10 years in, I am finally able to meet my practice members where they are at with their own health beliefs. I can lead them gently up the steps to embracing vitalistic principles. First, however I needed a fellow chiropractor to reach out and do that for me. Not through judgement or challenge, but through understanding and keen questioning, so that I could discover the answers that felt true for me. The result was to explode my business, expand my mind and spirit, and allow myself a life and a career that fills me with satisfaction and happiness. In turn, this allows me to serve my clients at a different level and show them the way to their own transformation. I will always be grateful to that mentor for her loving gift of walking me along the path: fierce, passionate and unwavering.

Whenever I see financial and spiritual freedom in this profession, I don't attribute it to confidence, sales-technique or good marketing. It's not insightful table talk, or no table talk, because two people who I greatly admire may do things very differently. What's special about them is that they are living true to their core values and have learned to become brave; they have pushed through some hardship and uncertainty and now live from the inside out. Certainty is inspiring, it's precious and it's not something you can effectively borrow; certainty that creates great change comes from the inside.

Living in Chiropractic is like walking across fire. We need to keep our energy higher than the fire, to get across unharmed. If you've ever done a fire walk, you will know that if you are not 100% in that belief, in that mindset, you will get burned. So, unless we are completely living into our own unique version of Chiropractic, we cannot possibly hold the energy, strength and courage required to bring the outer world on this journey with us. We give up, we get confused, exhausted and burn out.

In this profession, our task is to fully introduce ourselves and our vision to the world, leaving it changed forever by what we know. This is how we enlighten our community and inspire action. Since we cannot contort ourselves to fit in with traditional medicalised care, I believe we can only create this change in our community by gaining their trust. Trust is much more easily gained and maintained when we are able to be congruent with who we truly are. When we unleash this true part of ourselves, we can give reason for others to push through their own discomfort, and change. Then we get to watch the world re-order in front of our eyes.

When an explorer goes into a new forest, they mark a tree. This is their "touch tree" that they can always return to. No matter which path they take, or how far down a track they travel, so long as they can find their way back to this particular tree, they will not get lost. The last decade of my career has been spent finding my own touch tree. After hundreds of courses, seminars and events, hours spent thinking, "I wish I was like this person or that person", I finally found my own certainty by realising that what I needed above all else was an answer from within. A touch-tree I could always return to, while I explored the forest. The ability to align with my own unique set of values, based on key chiropractic principles. This allowed me to change everything about my technique, my clinic set-up, my values, my approach and change them back again without hesitation. It was painful, but each step was always worth it, because it was true for me. How could I know what was right? It went like this:

Moment of uncertainty arises.

Breathe, turn inward, connect.

Feel around for innate.

Do the next right thing, without apology.

Repeat.

Our goal however, should never be to remain the same, but to live in such a way that each moment, encounter, conversation, relationship and challenge becomes the material we use to change and re-invent. Pain and discomfort are often the fuel for this change; challenging our thinking and pushing through the resistance and fear. I often felt sick and fearful at the expected rejection from my community. What drives me ever-forward is the knowledge that, no matter what the outcome, if change is made for the right reasons, it's going to teach me something valuable. This is why we must never stop striving to become a better version of ourselves.

The personal gift of Chiropractic is to continue becoming truer, more beautiful versions of ourselves, again and forever. When we reflect the world that lives within us, we can change the world outside us. We are never "done", there is always more. By never holding too tightly to a single existing idea, opinion or identity, we can keep emerging new and more true. This is how we can travel deeper into the gifts of mind-body coherence and change how we relate to the world. This is truly connecting man the physical, to man the spiritual.

Once we begin to understand what does and does not fit with our values, we can also check that they still serve us. Since innate intelligence is specific, personal and ever-changing, we must consistently connect to this part of ourselves and course-correct. In every uncertain moment, turning inward, connecting with innate, and being brave in our action. When we learn to find the joy in uncertainty and change, we experience work and life at a different level. We are no longer divided by what we feel and know on the inside, in relation to what we say and do on the outside. Instead, we find ease through simply knowing we are taking that next step with a guaranteed learning experience at the end.

When you live within your values, some will recognise and respect your courage, while others may turn against you. This should not concern you, because you are serving exactly as you are meant to be. You can relax and know that those who you draw into your life are truly your people, while those who turn away simply leave more space for the ones who love you. You will never be forced to hide or act in order to keep people in your life, if you don't hide or act to get them there in the first place. When you are integrated, you have integrity.

While I truly believe that each precious person in this profession is right to express themselves in line with their beliefs, I hope of course they remain open-minded. This is how we can work to find our similarities rather than our differences. This is how we can walk down the staircase to someone else and help them up onto the next step. We can offer them the Celtic prayer of approach:

I honour your Gods,
I drink at your well,
I bring an undefended heart to our meeting place,
I have no cherished outcomes
I will not negotiate by withholding, and
I am not subject to disappointment.

In essence, I am not so tied to my need to persuade you that I cannot listen. I don't aim to fight or judge you. I am simply open to the dialogue. I am so certain of my truth and my experience that I want to sit with you and find the common ground, so that together, as a profession, we can create great change in the world.

So, I urge you to commit to yourself; that you will never again stay in a practice, a room, a conversation, relationship or institution that requires you to abandon yourself. When your innate tells you the truth, you accept it. Through the burning of old beliefs, we are reborn into new life-giving experiences. When we pay this lesson forward, mustering all our strength, patience and resilience, we can help others on their own journey. This will change not only their life, but the lives of those around them.

For this reason, we are called to be brave.

Wisdom #6

Laurence Tham DC

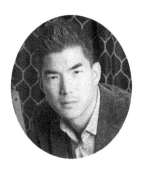

Laurence is a highly acclaimed and sought-after business coach for chiropractors worldwide. His passion and focus are the psychology of human behaviours, communications and potentials. His aim is to help chiropractors align their practices to their true selves and amplify their businesses with the latest marketing strategies.

Laurence has one of the largest family practices in Perth, Western Australia and is also co-host of The Wellness Guys Podcast and co-founder of a podcast network which hosts over 20 health and wellness podcasts.

The Journey of you

Chiropractic is stronger when individual chiropractors become more aligned with themselves and learn to AMPLIFY their voices. Collectively, we have the power to shift the consciousness of the world through our own practices. But it will take individual chiropractors to find their identities, to lift this profession to the next level.

Here are 3 key mindsets that I believe individual chiropractors can embrace to make this a reality.

Swim your own race

There is something magical about the Olympics. The plethora

of human emotions you get to experience from the highest of highs, to the lowest of lows. On the world stage, it is the ultimate display of preparation, passion and purpose.

In the 2016 Rio Olympics, I remember watching swimmer Katie Ledecky, a 19-year-old American, break her own world record by 1.91 seconds. Within the first 100 metres, it was clear she was in a class of her own. She was miles ahead of the entire race (winning the race by a margin of 4.77 seconds over the silver medallist).

During the race, I couldn't help but think, "What goes through your mind, during the race, if you are Katie Ledecky?" "What are the other swimmers, who are chasing Ledecky, thinking?"

Ledecky was clearly multiple body lengths ahead of her closest rival. Still, with a distance of 400 metres of swimming, there is only one thing you can think... SWIM YOUR OWN RACE. There is nothing else. It was just about her and the clock (and her own world record that she was chasing down).

But what if you were one of the other 7 competitors in that final?

I am sure there is a point in the race when you know that you can't catch up and you won't win. Mentally you'd have to switch your focus from chasing Ledecky to swimming your own race.

There is no other way.

We ultimately want what our friends or colleagues have. We want the life of the people we deem successful. We want to have what they have and do what they do. We chase and chase for those things, thinking that this will bring us more joy and happiness.

The moment you do this, you descend down a rabbit hole

of chase, without even asking why? It is easy to find yourself following everyone else - starting, building and buying a practice(s). Goals of seeing 200, 300, 400 patients a week. But is this what you want?

When I achieved all of the above, I found it didn't fulfil me. The chase pulls us away.

Away from what we truly want.

Away from what ultimately makes us happy.

Away from the true version of ourselves.

What we are chasing is someone else's dream.

And during the chase, we often lose sight of...

WHERE we are, WHAT we want, and WHO we are.

It is important to find mentors or people you admire... but not to imitate. I am not them, and they are not me.

As Oscar Wilde said, "*Be yourself. Everyone is already taken.*"

Staying in your own lane and swimming your own race is hard work. It's hard not to look over to see what others are doing. It is easy to want what others have, that you lack. It is easy to be unsatisfied with your own lack of progress, compared to others.

"*Success is peace of mind which is a direct result of self-satisfaction in knowing you made an effort to do your best, to become the best that you are capable of becoming*" - basketball coach John Wooden.

This is easy to say. The hard part is being honest with ourselves on the following question:

"Is this the best I've got?"

Only you can answer that, because at the end of the day there is no competition in life other than the competition with yourself. That is success.

Passion and Process

Many of us are told to follow our passions, yet many of us struggle much of our lives to discover what our passions are. This is because we define passion incorrectly.

I thought passion meant something you loved. Something you defined as your purpose. And to an extent, this is true. But it is not the definition of "passion".

Passion isn't something you find outside of yourself. Passion never comes from something you haven't done, or discovered. Passion can only be developed when you find something that you are willing to suffer for. Because the Latin root word of passion means "to suffer". As in Christianity, Passion of Christ means the suffering of Christ.

Your passion is something that you are willing to work for, grind for, die for. And you only discover this by putting in the time. This is known as "the process".

"The vision of a champion is someone who is bent over, drenched in sweat at the point of exhaustion when no one else is watching." - Anton Dorrance

In the small country town of Bowral, Australia, a young 9-year-old boy spent his after-school hours playing solitary games he created. One of these games was throwing a golf ball with one hand, against a corrugated water tank, while holding a cricket stump (not bat) in the other hand. The small ball would bounce off the water tank in unpredictable ways, and he would try to hit the ball with the cricket stump before it went past him.

To achieve this he needed discipline, creativity and incredible hand-eye coordination. Years and years of this one simple game, and this boy became known to the world as the greatest cricketer of all time, Sir Donald Bradman. Bradman had a Test batting career average of 99.94, which is considered to be the greatest achievement by any sportsman of any professional sport.

This is the Process.

The Process is a path in the pursuit of your goals/dreams. It is working the fundamentals instead of chasing shiny new objects, tactics and distractions. The Process is putting the 10,000 hours into mastering a particular skill, service or profession. It is to value learning, over anything else.

It is spending hours developing your muscle memory and speed on your adjustments. It is the willingness to practice your communication in telling the chiropractic story. It is producing video after video just to get better or the desire to write those blogs or delivering talks repeatedly until you become more comfortable with doing them.

This is the Process. It is the unspectacular preparation that no one sees, which creates spectacular achievement that everyone praises.

The Process ultimately creates your Passion. Passion leads you to Mastery. And Mastery defines you.

Find the Others

Michael Jordan was a master.

He is often viewed as one of the greatest basketball players of all time. He won multiple scoring titles, MVPs (most valuable player awards), and many individual accolades that have made him one of the greatest athletes ever. One of the most significant achievements was winning 6 NBA titles while playing for the Chicago Bulls in the 1980s and 1990s.

Michael Jordan was a phenomenal athlete. He worked harder than any other player and became a master of his craft because of the Process. But his individual achievements couldn't win him the elusive NBA championships all by himself.

It wasn't until another master coach and mentor, Phil Jackson, came along and told Michael that needed to trust and work with his teammates. He convinced Michael that in spite of his individual talent and skills, he could not win without his teammates.

Once Michael Jordan understood this, he began to pass. He began to trust and rely on his teammates like Scottie Pippen and Dennis Rodman to be the best versions of themselves. And as a team, they became world champions, 6 times over.

When I first took my oath at graduation "to do no harm", I was inspired to dedicate my life to serving others, to impact communities and somehow change the world.

In my early years, I was idealistic and driven with a purpose. But as time went by, life got in the way. Life tends to throw obstacles to challenge us, distract us from our path and test us to see if we are committed. I have failed these commitments many times over. But an internal unease always brings me back. It begins to question my sense of direction and eases me back towards the path of service.

When I was in my late 20s, I felt that I could accomplish this alone. I just needed to persevere, work and try harder. But as I grew older, I realised that it is about finding "the others".

The others who believe in what you believe in. The others who are as weird as you are. The others who are as passionate as you are. The other masters. Finding the others will help your cause. They help accelerate your impact by collaborating your strengths.

This allows you to stay in your lane, doing what you do best.

The others come in many forms.

They are our mentors, coaches and fellow collaborators.

They are clients, our team members and business partners.

Finding the others requires you to find yourself.

To know yourself.

And be yourself.

(Otherwise, they can't find you.)

Swim your own race.

Focus on your process.

Find the others.

Tom Waller MChiro, DC

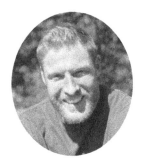 *Tom Waller DC is a full-time chiropractor and coach. He practices in Lincoln, UK alongside his wife Dr Sarah, in their busy family practice. Tom also runs a successful and bespoke coaching business for chiropractors and health professionals looking to bring more fulfilment to their bottom line.*

He is an international speaker, radio contributor and has held the position of Vice President of the United Chiropractic Association.

You are what you choose

"Chiropractic is a philosophy, science and art of all things natural." Defined in Stephenson's textbook and one of the original teachings in Chiropractic, this is what Chiropractic is. Nothing else.

However, what I would like to do is expand upon this for you, outside of chiropractic and inside your being. You may be reading this as a chiropractor, a student of Chiropractic or indeed a person who has no idea about Chiropractic. Wherever you find yourself reading this, what I want to share with you goes much deeper than the philosophy of this great profession. It is about you and your soul, your reason for being and how you choose to show up in this world.

The average human being has just 30,000 days on this planet. Think about that for a minute, just thirty thousand days! Now take your age, multiply it by 365 and take the number you get and subtract that from 30,000. What now?

I say this not to panic you but to enthuse you. Your time in the physical form, in the body you inhabit, is limited. And yes, we can utilise Chiropractic and other health benefits to give us more time. But what I would challenge you to do is really use your time purposefully. Your soul has chosen to inhabit the body you are reading this book from. Your soul is what gives you drive and direction, and your soul is the thing that will continue once this body stops.

The philosophy, science and art of life are how we choose to show up in life. If there is one teaching I can give you, it is to explore your philosophy and art more congruently. If we choose to live our true authentic philosophy the way we see the world, in our true authentic artistic way, then the time we have will be more fulfilling. We will be more present, we will have better connections and we will grow and deepen our soul. So that when the science of our physical body stops, our soul may continue with greater purpose in the world that awaits it.

While this book is full of great teachings and wisdom,

there is no more you really need to learn in life. It is not about discovering something new; it is about discovering what is already within you.

And the place to start is with your philosophy, your values. What do you truly believe and enjoy in life? Often we confuse our "values" with "social idealisms". These are actions and ways of being that we have been conditioned to believe are us because they are right and proper, because our father or teacher told us so. The simplest way to discover if what you are thinking is truly your value or a social idealism, is to listen to the little voice in your head, but only listen out for these two words: "should" and "must". These are the prefixes for all social idealisms. The one that gets people the most is the notion that they "should be a family man/woman", when their actions speak nothing of the sort. Spending time away and on other projects and distractions. This is not to say you do not love your family, they are simply not your highest value. Your highest value may indeed be the work or vocation that you choose, the byproduct of which serves your family.

But if you continue to tell yourself you are a family man and yet spend no time with family, incongruency will build, your actions and values will not align and this will breed destruction in your soul, your happiness and your relationships. Having the courage to self-inspect your values is grand. This self-discovery process is often uncomfortable but the ease and clarity that waits on the other side is remarkable.

Then take these values and find your way to bring them to the world. What is your art and your gift? What are you good at and what do you love to do? If you are reading this, it is quite possible you are a chiropractor and that you are good at it. Do you love it? Is it all that you want to do? Are there aspects of it you do just to please another soul, or are you in love with all that you do? The common example of this is the business aspect of practice and indeed the need within Chiropractic to acquire new customers and patients. Yes, you need to do this, but do you love to do this? Or does your gift and art lie in taking care of those people once under care? If so, be strong enough to admit that. Then find a way to work with others whose gifts and arts complement yours. Someone who is a great orator, who brings the masses to you but has no interest in delivering the care process. This is the symbiosis to be found in the universe once all our souls are congruent and aligned.

In this journey to discover ourselves, what I call "finding you", we need both courage and integrity. Courage to be who we are and the integrity to hold the promise to no one else other than ourselves, to show up as that person each and every day.

In Chiropractic, BJ Palmer was a great example of this. He chose to do what he wanted to do in life. He did not adapt to another person's word or philosophy, he stuck to his. He used his art and flair to bring it to the world and was not ashamed to do so. He even rode around town on an elephant and set up his own radio station. This confidence and integrity allow us to detach ourselves from the outcome, to remove the fear of judgment and do it anyway.

This selfishness allows us to be selfless. Selfishness in the pursuit of true passion and soul purpose is what we are here for. Our ability to discover our soul, to work through our limitations and to give love and meaning to our lives, brings love and meaning to the world.

So, when you choose to be a chiropractor, when you choose

to be successful, when you choose to do anything in life, that is your science. Know it, study it, perfect it but do not compromise your delivery of it. For that is your art.

Explore your philosophy. Find you and live a congruent life. Marry your values with your actions and take those actions daily to show up as the most authentic and genuine version of yourself possible.

My hope as you read this book is that you absorb all and learn; challenge everything; understand it all but never know it all. Mix it with your unique gifts so that we all may go out into the world with more passion, more purpose, and deeper, richer souls. So that those precious days we have become purposeful and leave a mark on history.

Wisdom #7

Craig Foote DC

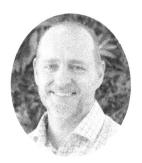 *Craig is a chiropractor of 21 years practice and lives in Perth, Western Australia. He is a co-founder of the Nervana Chiropractic Group and has a thriving practice in Perth's inner north suburbs. He has run multiple practices, trained successful associates and won awards for service to his community.*

Craig has been on the board of the Australian Spinal Research Foundation since 2011 and in that time he has helped direct more than $800,000 of investment into chiropractic research. He has been the president for the past 5 years. Craig is also a coach with Chiropractic Flight School, has 15 years' experience coaching and is a frequent guest lecturer at NZCC.

The surprising experience that changes everything

It is no small feat to shift a person from one paradigm to another, but that is what our job is, as a chiropractor. The greatest gift that we can give a person is the Big Idea. The concept that a person's body has an inherent ability to heal without interference. The risks are high. Do the right thing and the health of this person and their family benefits for life. Fail to help them shift and you commit them to a lifetime of health disempowerment and reliance on a failing, sickness-focused system.

On being asked to contribute to this project, I considered the many different lessons I have learnt over the years. I wanted to play just a small part in helping you in your practice to have a greater impact on the people that you see. I want the people that you care for to appreciate you for the wonderful and powerful person that you are. The sacrifices that you have made, the challenges that you have faced and most importantly the role that you and your unique skills and training may play in their lives.

As a chiropractic coach since 2003, there have been so many times where chiropractors have asked me, "Why don't my patients just get it?" The "it" refers to people choosing ongoing chiropractic check-ups in conjunction with a healthy lifestyle. How do we facilitate someone shifting from a paradigm that they have likely had their whole life, over to one that places self-empowerment and chiropractic at its centre?

Let's think like the "Average Joe" for a moment.

If you have a foot issue you see a podiatrist. A toothache, you see a dentist. A bowel issue, a gastroenterologist. If you are having back pain, you'd see your GP, a physio and if that doesn't work a chiropractor.

When a person decides to see a chiropractor, they are pre-loaded with previous experiences. These previous experiences then determine their expectations. It would be safe to assume that Joe has a pre-determined expectation of "once I'm out of pain the problem is gone". That is how it works with other professions, so why would Chiropractic be any different?

People entering your practice will either have a firm idea of the role that you should have in their health journey OR they have no idea at all and are genuinely seeking guidance. The guidance-seekers are clearly much more open to direction with their health and so from a paradigm shift, we are almost starting with a blank canvas, as their previous health paradigm has failed them somehow.

Joe is not one of those and he's just turned up at your practice. He's a patient who has firm beliefs as to how you can best serve him. Joe may say things like;

"I just need you to crack my back."

"Could I get you to have a look at my shoulder, it's been a bit sore."

"I know my body,"

Does this sound familiar? What do you do if what you offer is not what the patient has in mind?

In response to being placed in an inappropriate category, most chiropractors respond as any knowledgeable expert would. Hit them with data! "If I just give them the research, the case studies, the before-and-afters, the health talks, the proof, then surely something will stick and they'll finally get it!"

As a chiropractic coach, and as a someone who has headed up one of the world's largest chiropractic research foundations investigating subluxation (the Australian Spinal Research Foundation), let me state for the record that the answer is a resounding "no".

You can't fill a glass that is already full.

We need to do things a little differently right at our first meeting, so we get placed into the right category as a trusted health advisor. That approach starts with using surprise to our advantage. When we encounter something that surprises us, whether it be an unsolicited gift, an award or recognition, a party or even a prank, we respond by consciously focusing on our surroundings. We become open to whatever is going on around us. Our neurology is often buzzing with the anticipation of, "what's next?"

Consider the first time you went to your favourite restaurant. You were likely blown away because you didn't know what to expect and so it surpassed your expectations. You probably remember what you ordered, the cocktail that you had and possibly even the name of the person who served you that night. I would almost guarantee that you told everyone who would listen about how good the restaurant was and why they should go!

It is with this in mind, that we need to prime our patients for the paradigm shift which is going to occur. Now, we don't have to deliver silver service to new patients as they come in, although that would indeed be both unexpected and memorable. Rather we need to use both relevant and surprising questions. Questions are powerful tools. The person who asks the questions, controls the conversation.

The previous experience a patient has had with other professions can be polarised and it essentially sets up their first interaction with you. Your job is to work out what the preceding experience has been and determine whether they are likely to place you into your desired category.

The easiest scenario to deal with is the situation where the patient has had a preceding appalling experience with someone different to you, and with that in mind, they are very open to what you have to contribute. The much more difficult situation is when the patient has placed a previous health professional up on an unattainable imaginary pedestal. That might be a previous chiropractor who has retired, an orthopaedic surgeon who did their knee surgery, or a physio who helped them for a time.

"He saved my life."

"She's won all these awards."

"He worked with the state football team."

The challenge with dealing with these is that there is no way you can reach the perceived pedestal heights that they have reached until you differentiate yourself from them.

Consider a standard question asked in any initial consultation:

"Have you seen someone about this before?"

The answer would be yes or no, followed closely by justification, excuses or story-telling as to what made them choose that path. Average Joe would expect that. Asking the obvious question brings with it expectation and preparation from the patient's point of view. Whereas if you asked the question, "So, when Dr. Smith did their neurological, orthopaedic and chiropractic examination, were the X-rays they took standing up or lying down?"

Suddenly we have identified a gap in their knowledge that they never knew existed. We just emptied a little out of their glass. With just one question we have opened their mind to the concept that maybe we are different to Dr Smith. That we may deserve our own unique pedestal or even that Dr Smith's pedestal isn't that high after all.

The questions that you ask need to both relevant and surprising to have the desired effect. If X-rays weren't appropriate, other questions could be:

"So, when the physio did all of these tests to what degree did they go through your results?"

"So, when they did their 6 monthly reviews, did they make any changes to what they were focusing on?

"So, when you had that accident as a child, how many days

were you under observation for in hospital?"

"So, when you say your child does high-level gymnastics, which chiropractor do you regularly get them to see?"

It is the realisation that their experience wasn't as complete as they thought it was, that begins the shift in their paradigm. This realisation only comes from surprise experience. Experience trumps information every time. Experience is memorable. Information and data are more likely forgotten. Back to the difference in paradigms. Probably the most common difference is the perceived length of time that issues have been present. In the medical model, unless it is considered insidious and serious, it commonly is only a problem once pain begins. In a chiropractic model we identify that there can be issues without pain or symptoms for many years, causing a myriad of local and global issues.

"Joe, often these subluxations can be present in the spine for many years prior to causing obvious neck and back pain. Have you ever had any falls, sporting injuries, car accidents or been knocked out as a child?"

Pre-framing the question opens their mind to the possibility that perhaps what they are experiencing as an adult has actually been there since they were a child. If we do find that it has been there since they were young, then common sense would indicate that a long-term problem requires a long-term solution. We don't know that at the first meeting, however it is better to keep that door open just in case.

What about the assessment of the patient? I see far too many chiropractors missing the opportunity to even pre-frame their initial assessment. They will often conduct a great assessment and get excellent information in the pursuit of best helping the patient. That said, if you were to ask the patient afterwards, "What happened?" Their response will often be "They got me to move and bend and checked my posture."

Let's flip that around and set up the assessment before we touch them.

"Joe, in a normal functioning spine, if we were to touch each part, there would be movement (joint springing) and no tenderness. On the other hand, if we were to find a subluxation it wouldn't move under my thumb (that's what I would feel) and it would also be very sensitive or tender to touch (that's what you would feel)."

Even if you did nothing else you could do a simple static palpation of the spine with a massive difference. Joe would be focused on every touch from you. He would feel as though he played a part and may even say things such as, "There's one!" Any low-level chit-chat would be gone, leaving behind a very quiet but focused examination.

Let's take this even further, again before you touch them. "Joe, if we were to find any subluxations, we would then need to assess their impact on the nerves. As you'd expect, normally these nerves control things equally on both sides, however with subluxations we would see that one side clearly isn't able to control things as easily when we compare it to the other side."

I cannot tell you how important it is to get Joe to be focused on the experience of the assessment BEFORE it happens.

Using the words; "Let's compare that to the other side" throughout your assessment will open Joe's mind to perhaps there's more going on here than what he first thought. What's more, no one has been as thorough as this before.

First impressions last. What foot we start off on sets us up for either success or failure. Just being under chiropractic care is not enough. Having your patients understand chiropractic and health principles and helping them implement them into their lives is a much better measure of success. To quote my late friend Dr David Russell, *"Chiropractic is a big F$%king deal."*

This is a big deal when you consider that we are attempting to shift their paradigm. Let's honour it by doing the best job we can as chiropractors.

Peter Kevorkian DC

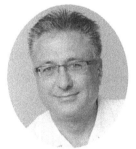

Peter and his wife Patti run a very special home/office practice which is considered the "standard" in family chiropractic care. Peter teaches internationally on chiropractic philosophy, children and Chiropractic, and family practice.

A proud father of two home-born children, Peter is President and instructor for the ICPA, former Chairman of Sherman College of Chiropractic and he serves on the board of the Massachusetts Chiropractic Society. He and his wife sponsor regular "Philosophy Nites" at their home, the longest continuous running group of its kind in the world.

Salutogenesis, Chiropractic Philosophy and Clinical Service

Salutogenesis is a term coined by Aaron Antonovsky nearly 40 years ago. The actual word means "giving birth to health". Antonovsky recognised that just because a person was successfully treated for medical conditions, it did not necessarily mean that they were healthier or well. Chiropractors have always promoted the fact that a healthy body is one that is functioning properly, and not necessarily one that is free of diagnosed conditions. Since the birth of our profession, chiropractors have understood that wellbeing is a natural and normal phenomenon. I would like to explore the concept of salutogenesis and how it interfaces with chiropractic practice and chiropractic philosophy.

The philosophy of chiropractic is based on a deductive reasoning, starting with an assertion (premise) that there is order and organisation in the universe. From that "Big Idea" we have created a profession that strives to improve the quality of life in people by reducing interferences to the human nervous system. The conservative faction of the chiropractic profession continuously asserts that we do not "treat" conditions, rather, we contribute to the wellbeing of people by adjusting spinal subluxations. This non-therapeutic focus has always lacked a word that could describe that focus. Salutogenesis may be that term.

The therapeutic focus is pathogenic. Pathogenesis (creation of disease) is the primary focus in the healthcare system. Case management is built upon diagnosis and treatment. Salutogenesis is the antagonistic term to pathogenesis. As a new term and new concept, the application of this approach is in the process of becoming defined in our culture. I believe that Chiropractic will be a major contributor to this approach in healthcare.

Antonovsky points out that there is a continuum in care from salutogenic (health-ease) to pathogenic (disease-ease).

Within the pathogenic approach, the care giver will diagnose, treat, and strive to cure. In this direction, a determinant is made of what is broken or dysfunctional and one strives to remove it or fix it. The case is managed based upon this dysfunction, and the person is dismissed once the condition is effectively treated and resolved. Within a salutogenic approach, a care giver will assess how they can intervene to improve the system. Most often the determinants for intervention are for wellbeing or vitality. In this model, a case is not necessarily managed, there is continued positive input into the system and the input can continue for a lifetime. Inputs such as eating wholesome foods, exercising regularly, and negotiating stressors through personal disciplines are examples of salutogenic input without necessarily "treating" a pathology. In a salutogenic model, the goal is to optimise the system and there is not necessarily a predetermined endpoint.

Chiropractic philosophy is underscored with a recognition that the body is a self-healing, self-regulating organism. The goal of chiropractic intervention is not to control, manipulate or manage the body. It is to honour the life process and give a positive input (spinal adjustment) to the body to allow ideal adaptability and functionality.

The interesting challenge on a philosophical and practice perspective in the context of salutogenesis, is the issue of vertebral subluxation. It is possible to view a subluxation as a condition that needs to be treated. There are many chiropractors who view a subluxation as a diagnosis upon which we develop a treatment programme to remove or eliminate. As a contrast, there are some who view a subluxation as a phenomenon that is held in the body as a result of the body being subjected to non-adaptable forces. They view the goal of the adjustment being not to treat or restore. It is to free and integrate.

There are 3 practice approaches that the chiropractor who exclusively analyses and adjusts subluxations can employ:

The first is to adjust vertebral subluxations with the intention of treating diagnosed conditions (eg adjust the atlas misalignment to treat headaches). The subluxation is viewed as an entity that needs to be removed (pathogenic) and it is causing some type of disorder or disease (pathogenic). This clearly fits within the pathogenic model of clinical intervention. This type of care is therapeutic in nature.

The second is to adjust vertebral subluxations with the intention of restoring spinal integrity either biomechanically or neurophysiologically (or both). This is done for the maximum adaptability of the physiology. The subluxation is looked at as a condition of the body that needs to be reversed and treated (pathogenic). The care of the person is salutogenic but the attention on the subluxation is pathogenic.

The third approach has the intention of giving positive input into the nervous system. The subluxation is viewed as a phenomenon. The adjustment does not "undo" the subluxation rather it allows the body to adapt that force and bring the body to a greater level of ease. This type of approach is salutogenic in both how the chiropractor addresses the subluxation and how the impact of the input is viewed on the physiology.

In all 3 approaches, the chiropractor holds the adjustment as the central point of care.

Antonovky's theory was based upon a person's use of coping mechanisms under times of stress. He termed this ability to cope as a "sense of coherence". Sense of coherence (SOC) is a theoretical formulation he created to explain stress in human functioning. The higher a person's sense of coherence, the better they can adapt to stressors. The sense of coherence has three components:

- Comprehensibility: a person's ability to understand what is happening in their life and predict what will happen in the future.
- Manageability: a person having the skills or the support or the resources to take care of things. They are in control of things in their life.
- Meaningfulness: a person feeling a sense of worthiness and fulfillment in their life. They care about what happens in their life.

From a philosophical standpoint, one would expect that a spine free of spinal subluxations would allow a person to have a greater sense of coherence. Research is beginning to suggest that this is true. Quality of life assessments (eg PROMIS-25) as well as other physiological tools (eg Heart Rate Variability) allow an objective measurement of aspects of SOC. As one receives regular chiropractic care there is an improved SOC.

Subluxation-centered chiropractic care is a unique tool in the healthcare system. It can not only show an increased sense of coherence through quality of life assessments and physiological metrics, the very nature of adjusting the subluxation phenomena lends itself clinically to an increased sense of coherence.

Adjusting spinal subluxations improves comprehensibility. When a subluxation is present, the brain cannot perceive the body or the environment. When the person is adjusted and there is less irritation on the spinal cord and nerves, comprehensibility increases. Hence, a person's SOC increases.

Adjusting spinal subluxations improves manageability. When a subluxation is present, the brain cannot control the body or the environment as well. When the person is adjusted and there is less irritation on the spine cord and nerves, manageability increases. Hence, a person's SOC increases.

When a chiropractor explains that the body is a self-healing, self-regulating system or that the body makes every drug or chemical that the body should need in a lifetime, we allow people to be reminded of how amazing the body is. We allow them to learn (or relearn) that their body (or that of their children) is their responsibly to care for. The body can be trusted. This may increase a person's meaningfulness and hence raise a person's SOC.

Although there is not a clear equal sign between Antonovsky's theories and ideas, and chiropractic philosophy and logic, there are many aspects that dovetail with each another.

I believe that the healthcare culture and the healthcare consumer are both awakening to a new paradigm. People are recognizing that treating conditions is a very small aspect of wellbeing. People want to contribute to their body functioning better by giving it positive input. Never before have more healthcare dollars been spent on whole foods, organic foods, personal growth experiences, health clubs and the like. People are ready to engage professionals to support their wellbeing and not just treat problems. More than ever before, people need to hear the chiropractic story. People need to have a more adaptive and resilient nervous system. People need to regularly engage in activities that offer positive input to their physiology. Consulting a care giver on a regular basis to maximize wellbeing and vitality is almost unheard of in any healthcare circles except for a vitalistic chiropractic practice. We have an opportunity to define this support with our ideals and our unique service.

Wisdom #8

Arno Burnier DC

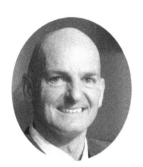

Arno Burnier DC is a Vitalistic Chiropractor with a handsome pedigree. A 1977 graduate of Sherman College of Chiropractic, he is the founder of MLS Seminars, ABC Seminars and Spinal Motion Palpation Seminars.

He practices from his home in Durango, Colorado and is married with two grown up children. Dr Arno is the founder and owner of the Café of Life Vitalistic Practice Model and is a world-renowned speaker on Chiropractic, also often advising colleges and helping chiropractors to find their own vision as a cofacilitator of THRIVE Seminars.

The power of the adjustment

Between the bird and the book, I follow the bird. Between theory and experience, I learn from the experience. It is said that one who learns things by experiences, increases knowledge. I was blessed and cursed by 2 opposite and extreme experiences in Chiropractic. They were to transform my life in a profound manner.

Chiropractic philosophy has always been my forte, love and passion. Yet I will put it aside for now, in order to share what I perceive to be of paramount importance.

Like most in Chiropractic, I had learned about subluxation. I had been exposed to many theories and models of subluxations. I also refused to believe blindly in the reality of subluxation. Its theories sounded plausible as well as fascinating. Could there really be a blockage to the expression of the life force, which is chi, light and spirit in the body? Could it be true that, if life force was released fully, one could experience the totality of one's innate expression? Could the transmission of innate forces indeed be interfered with and possibly released through adjustments?

Philosophically it all sounded amazing, full of possibilities. Yet in the reality of practice and of being adjusted, I did not experience nor witness the promise of the philosophy.

Yes, I felt more relaxed, more balanced, maybe even more attuned to myself, with a quieter mind for few moments following an adjustment. I could even feel more ease in my being and trusting it facilitated proper function.

Yes, I saw great outcomes in practice. At times, puzzling and amazing results. Yet, no, I had not seen the fullness of what the philosophy stated the adjustment ought to deliver. Like most chiropractors, I lived in trust and doubt when it came to the reality of subluxation. I was not an evidence-based DC. To some degree I admired and resented those who lived by evidence-based only. Admired them for seeking evidences as to the existence of subluxation and resented them for challenging or denying the philosophy that I love so much, since we could not accumulate sufficient evidences to prove its veracity. Lack of evidence is not evidence of lack. That always kept me in trust of the truth of the philosophy.

In the mid 1980s I was at a chiropractic convention at the Waverly in Atlanta, Georgia. A woman named Helene Ginian came to me during the Saturday evening banquet. I had met her in the past. She knew who I was and my notoriety within chiropractic circles. She asked me to step out of the banquet room, wanting to talk to me. I acquiesced. Outside the noisy room, she implored me to get adjusted by Donny Epstein, DC. I had taught philosophy at Donald Epstein's seminars for few years, so I knew him. What he was doing and was up to, I had no idea.

So, on the pleading of Helene, I decided to check things out. After the banquet Donald Epstein was adjusting in the vendor's area. There was an open adjusting table. I sat on it and waited for him. He came behind me, felt the tone of my body and neuro-spinal system. I lay down. He proceeded to adjust me. Within minutes it was over. I got up, thanked him and walked back to my hotel room settling for the night. On my way back, I thought, "What was the big deal? What was Helene making such a fuss about?" It felt fine, but no different to other adjustments.

The next morning, he was adjusting again. I sat on an open table. Again, he came behind me to feel the tone. I turned my head to look at him and for some reason said, "Take me home". I lay face down on the table. He took few gentle contacts, adjusted a few vertebrae structurally and took another gentle contact near my sacrum. Suddenly I felt an enormous concentrated energy building up at the base of my spine, the intensity of it building up so fast that it felt like a dam was going to burst.

The next thing I knew, I let out a roaring primal scream. I felt like a rocket had been placed inside my rectum, fired up and launched upward, travelling at lightning speed up my spine to explode into my brain. The next instant, my brain was illuminated by white light and my entire body was pulverized and permeated by white light. I no longer had any perception of my physical body.

I was pure vibrating energy and light. The only other way I can attempt to convey the experience, is that I felt I was plugged into 100,000 watts of electricity with no discomfort, just pure ecstasy. I was bathed by the light, in total bliss. There is nothing, not a thing, which could have been added or subtracted from the experience to make it any better. Anything done thereafter would have taken away from the blissful state.

It is only years later reading David Hawkins book, *The I of the Eye* where he shared his experience of enlightenment that I realised I had experienced that same state of being. I could have written his account myself, it was identical.

For the next 3 months, I sustained that blissful state of being. I had no desire to speak, silence felt so complete. I practiced in nearly total silence. I was compelled to meditate morning and evening. I could no longer eat meat. The first bite I took became like chewing gum; I just could not swallow it. I became celibate, having zero sexual desires. These changes came from within. All my energy had risen to the higher realms. I had clear immediate knowing of people's state and past.

I witnessed spontaneous healing in my practice like never before. I could hardly touch people, my hands were so full of light; they would have instantaneous transformation, bursting into tears, emoting, releasing stored emotions, traumas and dampened energy or have their symptoms disappear in a matter of minutes. In an instant, "Coca-Cola glasses" were no longer needed for a 13-year-old girl named Selena. Amy's years of anorexia vanished in one visit, never to return. Mary became a horse whisperer the day of her first adjustment.

Another woman emitted the gurgling sound of drowning while getting adjusted. We found out later from her mother that she had nearly drowned as a baby in a tub. My sister-in-law Kelly was "dead" for few minutes on the table, no pulse, nor breathing. The apnoea lasted long enough for me to call Donald Epstein asking him what I should do. Following his guidance, I held a posterior axis contact and she came back to life. She had been a stillborn and had had to be resuscitated. People were reliving, releasing and clearing past trauma stored in cellular memories.

Over the years I have shared my experience on chiropractic public speaking platforms. Often people in the audience came to me afterwards. They shared that they too had had similar experiences of being adjusted by either Donald Epstein or by the DCs he had taught. As it turned out, thousands of lay people and hundreds of students and DCs received those adjustments during the mid 1980s.

One may ask: "What happened? Is this still available?" The answer is no, not that I know of. Donald Epstein was attacked and vilified by our profession. State Boards prohibited the practice of Network Spinal Analysis. Most DCs could not handle witnessing such power. Their egos couldn't handle it. They could not comprehend what they were seeing. So, he "shelved" the adjustment. That window of time closed for now.

From this experience I knew, beyond the shadow of a doubt, that subluxations are a reality within the neuro-spinal system. What they are, what actually is taking place neurologically, I have no idea. But one thing I know for sure is that the light or spirit in my being was blocked, unbeknown to me, and was released in its totality by the adjustment.

Sub-lux-ation equals less light in expression. An amazing choice of a word by the Palmers that encompasses the possibility of, less than a luxation, to fit the mechanical world view of the time, as well as, less than light in expression, to fit the energetic, vitalistic present worldview.

Again, for the subluxation deniers with all the respect and rights they deserve, lack of evidence is not evidence of lack. My experience along with thousands of others, validates the existence of subluxations.

It is not because science has not yet caught up to explain what is happening that things are not happening. Subluxation is a reality. Our present capacity to remove them is still in its infancy. The art of chiropractic is young and new. What is 100 years? Where was medicine after 100 years? Where was the wheel after 100 years?

What took place during those magical years in the mid 1980s is a peep preview into the upcoming maturity of the art of adjusting. It showed the potential of the adjustment to release life force. It is the promise of a bright future for our profession as long as we persist on the path set out by the philosophy and science of chiropractic. We need to grow and mature as practitioners to handle responsibly, this kind of capacity and power. We are not there yet.

During that time, I brought my wife Jane, my mother and father in-law, Helen and Bill, my three sisters in-law, Kelly, Mary Ellen and Patty and my brother in-law, Russ to Donald Epstein. All had similar experiences.

Jane and I went to visit Donald Epstein's office in Bellmore, New York, numerous times. What we saw during those visits was nothing short of the miracles written about in the bible. Surgical osseous fusion of joints in the foot breaking loose by the light with full motion restored. A concentration camp survivor in her eighties, who could not walk since childhood due to damage inflicted by Nazis, standing up without support and walking, then slow dancing with joy. We saw black smoke coming out of a man's mouth, while getting adjusted. He had been in an airplane fire years before and had had respiratory problems ever since. An elderly woman spontaneously adopted challenging yoga postures as the body was driving the released life force where it was needed, for healing.

Indeed, the capacity of the body to heal is beyond our wildest imagination when the spinal channel is fully open. In 2018 I went to Brazil to teach an adjusting seminar. Jane and I had lunch with a DC who came from Argentina to help with the seminar. He appeared to have psychic abilities. He shared with us things about Jane's dead mother that no one but us could possibly know. It lead me to trust him. He offered to adjust me. I received a brutal, violent, disconnected and angry lumbar adjustment. Immediately I felt damaged.

The pain I experienced shot through my back and leg. For months afterwards I could not sit without extreme pain. I spent six months eating all my meals standing. I avoided sitting as much as possible. Over time, things slowly improved. Yet I still experience chronic nerve pain in my right leg and foot. I feel like my foot is a cement block. At times it feels like a blowtorch is pouring fire on my foot, my ankle feels as though it is in a vice, being crushed. At times walking is impossible as I cannot even place my right foot on the ground, the pain is so severe. My leg and my life have atrophy. I am limited in the distance I can walk, the length of time I can sit. I look for reprieve by lying down and look forward to the nights in bed.

Why is it so important for me to share these experiences, that I would forfeit writing about chiropractic philosophy?

Because I want students and DCs alike to know the possibilities of the power of an adjustment: one to bring enlightenment, the other to cripple a life and a body.

One moment of unconsciousness, one instant of disconnection, not being attuned to the being on the table, not being present, not being clear with oneself can cause an adjustment to be devastating to a person's life. Being fully in the heart, fully conscious, aware and present, connected to one's soul, in the spirit of service, could cause light to be released in the body bringing the experience and state of enlightenment, if the proper skills are available. That is the power we hold in our heart, soul and hands.

Amazingly, Head-Heart-Hands is a symbol for chiropractic. No one can take those experiences away from me. From them, I gain knowledge as to the reality of subluxation and the potential of the adjustment. Adjusting is to be taken seriously, with utmost reverence. It is a sacred act to touch, access, and adjust the most core and sacred system within a human being. There is nothing more core than the neuro-spinal system in the body.

With knowledge, comes responsibility. Having read what I just shared imparts you the reader with responsibilities. We, as a profession, along with our teaching institutions, must train our students with the sacredness, rigor, discipline and professionalism that are called for to respect such a powerful art, the art of adjusting. As BJ Palmer stated: "*The sole purpose of the adjustment, is to unite the spiritual with the physical.*" I now know the truth of that statement. I can attest to its veracity from my own experience.

Ben Purcell DC

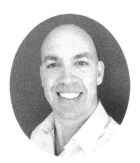

Dr Ben Purcell completed his Master of Chiropractic through Macquarie University in 2008. As a younger man, Ben sustained multiple injuries playing rugby and horse riding causing episodes of debilitating neck and back pain. Then at 23 he worked for a Chiropractor in Sydney and finally found relief through Chiropractic Adjustments. This experience combined with helping people in a clinical setting inspired him become a Chiropractor. As well as being a dedicated family man, Ben runs a very successful practice in Bathurst Australia and he also mentors other Chiropractors on behalf of Dr Don and Brandi MacDonald's Vitaly Engine.

Care Planning: Salutogenic vs Pathogenic Model

What we believe matters! What we believe impacts all decisions in our daily life. For Chiropractors what we believe, what we value and how we communicate our message in daily practice is directly related to what we believe Chiropractic to be, otherwise known as our Chiropractic premise. Often our premise is based on how Chiropractic has helped ourselves personally, then is heavily influence by where we studied and by our mentors.

From what I can see there are two ends of the scale for our premise. Neither are good or bad, better or worse, they just are and the quicker you can figure out where your premise lies then the better you will understand yourself, your message and why your practice looks the way it does.

The two ends of the scale are the salutogenic philosophy

and the pathogenic philosophy of health. The philosophy or model that you "believe" to be true will permeate though every single interaction in daily practice; all your conversations, your language, your procedures, your staff training, your marketing and most of all what you recommend as a schedule of care for the people you serve. I believe nothing is truer than when it comes to care planning, and in the wise words of Brandi MacDonald "you will promise what you premise"!

To take this conversation further we need some definitions:

Salutogenesis

Salutogenesis is a term coined by Aaron Antonovsky, a professor of medical sociology. The term describes an approach focusing on factors that support human health and well-being, rather than on factors that cause disease. More specifically, the "salutogenic model" is concerned with the relationship between health, stress, and coping. Antonovsky's theories reject the "traditional medical-model dichotomy separating health and illness". He described the relationship as a continuous variable, what he called the "health-ease versus dis-ease continuum".

Pathogenesis

The pathogenesis of a disease is the mechanism that causes the disease. The term can also describe the origin and development of the disease, and whether it is acute, chronic, or recurrent. The word comes from the Greek pathos and genesis. Types of pathogenesis include microbial infection, inflammation, malignancy and tissue breakdown. Most diseases are caused by multiple processes. For example, certain cancers arise from dysfunction of the immune system. Often, a potential etiology is identified by epidemiological observations before a pathological link can be drawn between the cause and the disease.

Why is this important when it comes to care planning?

If your belief is that we are treating a pain or a condition, then your premise will fall heavily to the pathogenic sided of the equation. If you believe that what you are doing is helping people express life to the greatest of their potential, then your premise will fall more so on the salutogenic side of the equation. It is my opinion that all Chiropractors fall somewhere between these two opposing philosophies and unless the Chiropractor can define where they sit then they will live with a degree of confusion in daily practice.

When referring to the pathogenic philosophy, the very nature of treating a pain or condition means that at some stage once that pain or condition has abated (if it ever does) then you as a practitioner will have to choose one of three courses of actions.

Option one: discharge the practice member from your care. They presented with neck pain, now do not have neck pain so you have fulfilled your agreement and your job is done.

Option two: find another pain or condition to treat. Engage a great deal of energy to "re-sell" the benefits of chiropractic care and your services for the new pain or condition, create a new agreement and hopefully have a chance to get on with the job. Once again when you have achieved your agreed goal you are back at the same position with the same three options.

Option three: move the practice member to some form of a "wellness" program of care. This option is dressed up in many forms and ultimately results in the chiropractor educating their patient as to the benefit of long-term care. Once again, the chiropractor must re-engage their sales strategies to create value for long term care.

From what I have observed many chiropractors have trouble defining a clear picture of "wellness". Is it that their practice members remain pain free? Move better? Think clearer? Digest better? What happens when life throws a curve ball at the practice member? What happens if all the original symptoms that were previously "fixed" returns? Does this mean you didn't fix the problem? Have you taken the practice member for a ride? Are you able to use objective measures to comfortable say that the practice member is living in a state of wellness and what does the schedule of care look like to keep them in that "state"?

I see and hear of many chiropractors following the age old "monthly" schedule of care for wellness without having a clearly defined guideline as to what "wellness" looks like and no clear justification as to why a monthly adjustment can fulfill the promise of their undefined wellness.

On the flip side Chiropractic and the salutogenic philosophy is all about the individual being more adaptable and resilient to their life experience. To support the practice member to a healthier state irrespective of their pain or condition and irrespective of where they are on the health continuum from extreme dysfunction/near death to optimal cohesion/expression of life. Under the salutogenic model Chiropractic is not trying to "fix" the practice members pain or condition. Under the salutogenic model Chiropractic is helping the individual express more of their functional and healing capacity, moving the practice member towards a more balanced and connected state by supporting their neurology through the Chiropractic adjustment.

This belief permeates through all interactions with the practice member. The initial consult requires more effort on behalf of the chiropractor and team to gather the required information to determine how efficient the individual's neurology is able to process their world. Some of the most powerful tests are the simplest known to science however when performed and communicated in context are supremely impactful. It is the communication of what we discover plus linking to the values of the practice member that holds a key in implementing the salutogenic model. To help move an individual from just wanting a "fix" to wanting to thrive.

The education process of a practice member towards a better state of health, healing, resilience and adaptability requires a great deal of energy and awareness from the chiropractor and their team. I use the "Hierarchy of Vitality" from Dr Don & Brandi MacDonald's The Vitality Shift communication program (which is where I was initially exposed to these concepts) to map out the stages of healing from a "stuck" state of physiology to a state of optimal expression. Not every person wants to move to an optimal state, some start the journey and life takes them another way and some due to the poor and damaged state of their system will never reach a state of optimal health however each person who enters a chiropractor's office who values optimising the practice members neurological capacity should be measurably healthier from the care they receive.

Under the salutogenic model of care the offer from the chiropractor is to test, measure and address the individuals state, not fix or treat a pain or condition. Often many pains and conditions resolve although this is never the promise. A care plan under the salutogenic model is a continual process and evolution that increases and decreases with the highs and lows of the practice members life.

Since I have employed the salutogenic philosophy into practice from late 2017 I have found myself and my practice to be lighter in energy, I am busier and more fulfilled, I also work with more clarity and passion.... why? I am helping people in the most honest way I know; I am helping people be better versions of themselves and sometimes they still have pain and still have their health conditions however they know, and I know that they are healthier as a result of the care they are receiving.

I believe one of greatest expressions of life for a human being is to live in a state of optimal cohesion with themselves and their environment; this is ultimately what I believe Chiropractic care brings to our communities and the people we serve.

Wisdom #9

Ryan Rieder MTech (Chiro), DC

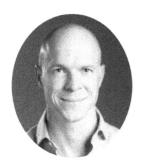

Ryan grew up and studied Chiropractic in South Africa. He and his chiropractor wife Natalie moved to the UK where he co-founded Hälsa Care Group which owns and operates 8 offices with over 100 team members.

Ryan is also the founder of DC Practice Growth and New Patient Avalanche System which helps chiropractors all over the world grow their practices with his tried-and-tested strategies. He is an international speaker and his book The New Patient Avalanche System is a #1 best-seller on Amazon.

You don't find Chiropractic, it finds you

Or at least that's my journey. There are 5 first-generational chiropractors in my family, my mother-in-law helps with our bookkeeping and my sister-in-law is a practice manager. To say we are all in, is an understatement. We have 8 practices and about 200,000 visits per year.

The truth is that the chiropractic profession is truly an entity that keeps on giving. It is no surprise that one of chiropractic's most famous quotes is BJ Palmer's, *"You never know how far reaching something you think, say, or do today, will affect the lives of millions tomorrow."*

These words point to a vision greater than us and also to a vision that we can never quite quantify. We could never sum up the effect chiropractic has on the planet and the impact it has on our lives as chiropractors!

Because of this wonderful profession, not only did I meet my wife with whom I have 2 beautiful children, both adjusted since birth, they also have had it instilled within them from an early age the understanding that, "what made the body, heals the body". My heart explodes every time my 3-year-old looks at a bump or bruise and says, "Don't worry Daddy, my body will heal itself."

There is something quite wonderful about instilling self-belief in a human being. That's really what Chiropractic is for me. The instilling or connecting the belief back in "self" and it is one of the most attractive philosophies I have ever come across.

Just take the fact that in my 10-year career we are averaging at least one chiropractic assistant per year going on to enrol to study chiropractic, let alone the many practice members who do. I don't know any profession that is capable of that.

There must be something to it

I can only speak for myself and my path but what I can tell you is that whenever I'm a bit lost, I can always rely on this wonderful profession to help me find my path.

At school I was a terrible student, only focused on sport. I was truly lost as to what my next step after school would be, until one day I discovered that my neighbour was going to study to become a chiropractor. At that point I had never even been to a chiropractor.

Intrigued, I set off to observe the local chiropractor without any pre-conceived ideas. And just like that within 30 seconds of being in that room, something happened. I saw happy smiley faces moving toward joy and that was me, hooked.

Motivation is much like staying clean. To stay clean, you need to cleanse daily; to stay motivated or on fire, you need to practice it daily or stay close to it!

Unfortunately, the fire is lacking in most educational environments, which was certainly the case for me. In fact, I had a lecturer look me in the eye in my final year and suggest I choose another career path because in his words, "It is too hard to make it."

Once again, I was lost and just before graduating I enquired about studying a post graduate medical degree, in essence, to become a medical doctor.

I needed to pay for this venture and figured that I would practice and study.

Once again chiropractic simply had to knock and pull me towards the truth. I remember walking into my first chiropractic job interview and again the overwhelming surge of smiley faces hit me within seconds. By the end of the shift, I was 'in'. It's the people that are touched by Chiropractic that guide me towards truth.

"Success in spite of us"

The simplicity of Chiropractic often stupefies those on the outside, and the concept of a sort of panacea through which all things are better, is something again that "just can't be."

Many from the outside would say that the catchphrase "Above, down, inside, out", is oversimplified, BUT it is simply perfect and can be applied to every single area of a person's life.

This profession has saved many lives: it has without a doubt saved mine. I am by virtue a simple entrepreneur. My modus operandi is to observe that which already works, and model it.

I think too many entrepreneurs take false credit for things that they "invented." Poppycock, I say.

While recently teaching a certain formula of success, a coach of mine told me that these formulae were not created but simply observed in "the successful" and then collated.

My favourite BJ Palmer story and subsequent favourite quote comes from a sort of folk tale. It is rumoured that BJ once said that, *"You could hit someone in the arse with a snow shovel and innate would use the force to reduce the subluxation and the body would heal."*

The reason that this is my favourite story is because I've always thought that talent was overrated and I often joke that I'm so lucky to have stumbled across a profession that just works.

Every adjustment delivered with the right intention works. Yes, the application of the adjustment, like any art, needs to be practiced and improved upon in the pursuit of perfecting one's craft.

In much the same way that any good diet or exercise moves the body towards a greater homeostasis and health, so too does any chiropractic adjustment.

Is it really that simple?

Luckily for you, yes, it is! Now you just need to TRUST more. Much like nature not needing more help but rather no more interference, so too does chiropractic not need anything MORE added to it.

BJ Palmer once said, *"So what Chiropractic does, is that it simply takes the handcuffs off Nature,"* as it were.

The truth is that it's often the chiropractor who simply needs to have the handcuffs of their educated mind taken off. I was once taught that fear is simply "lacking in faith".

This is not some esoteric finding of faith, but simply the understanding that one need only observe, to see that not only does chiropractic "work", it always works. We are blessed to be in this wonderful profession!

Conor Ward MChiro, PG Cert, DC

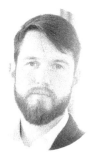

Since qualifying in 2008, Conor has spent much of his career working for Halsa Care Group, one of the largest providers of chiropractic services in the UK. He spent 2014 in Peru at Centro Quiropractico Schubel, the largest chiropractic company in South America. Conor believes chiropractors must play a key role in reversing the trend of lifestyle-induced illnesses. His natural talent for innovation and networking has led to him helping the entire profession in spreading this message, through his leadership group The Lions of Chiropractic, with an annual conference and regular online webinars.

Three brutal truths that are difficult to admit

It is easier to dwell in the comfort zone of light conversations, than to delve into the darker truths. If you intend to have an impact on the world it is imperative that you put life in perspective; that you boldly step into the dark, in order to grow. This helps you gain the wisdom to realise your true potential and live life to the full. This piece will uncover some brutal truths that are difficult to admit, regarding happiness, mortality and knowledge.

Your Material Wealth Will Not Make You A Happier Person

Modern society instils a drive for the accumulation of status symbols and the appearance of a perfect life. This drive is fuelled by never-ending marketing messages and comparing our lives to people we follow on Instagram. There is nothing wrong with enjoying the finer things in life, in fact I encourage you to do so, but with the conscious realisation that lasting happiness lies within you. It is related to the relationships you forge, finding ways to contribute or working within what you consider to be your purpose.

Self-awareness is the key to a fulfilled life. Understanding who you are, what drives you and how to overcome traumas, is a lifelong quest. The challenge is that we develop narratives in our head about what we think will make us happy, passed down from our families, our friends or society. We say things like, "I'll be happy when I get married..." or "When I earn X amount..." The reality is that happiness is always present in your life; self-awareness helps you connect to it and allows it to flow though you. The first and most important relationship to improve is the one you have with yourself. All the external love in the world will not help you find happiness until you cultivate internal self-love. It is also important to understand that you cannot make everybody happy and if you try, you will lose yourself. Start respecting your values, principles, and autonomy.

The longer you spend pretending that the ultimate truths do not exist, the more time you waste chasing a shadow of your true identity. You are the author of your own life, stop looking for sympathy and start creating the life story you want to read. Now is the only time that matters, not what happened in your past and not what might happen in the future. Time is your most valuable commodity and you have both the power and responsibility to decide what you do with it. Ambition is nothing without the action steps and the consistent work required to make things happen. Investing in yourself is not selfish. In fact, it could be the most important thing you do to stretch yourself and grow your life to the biggest it can be.

None of us can be perfect and in our attempts at perfectionism we often create unrelenting inner critics that tear us apart inside. Appreciation for ourselves and our achievements allows us to fight back against that negative voice, amplifies intuition, and challenges unrealistic standards. The irony is that we try to hide or overcompensate for our perceived flaws, but having the courage to allow ourselves to be vulnerable with people is a real strength that creates strong and meaningful connections.

If you have a damaged relationship with someone significant in your life, it may be up to you to rise above the past transgressions to move forward. How you react matters, so train yourself to respond in a way that creates a better outcome. Aim to always act in the kindest way for you and them. If you feel you have done all you can to repair a relationship, let it be ok for you to allow that person to pass from your day-to-day life or create a situation where they can have the least negative impact on you. You should aim to gravitate towards people who celebrate you for who you are, point out when you are being ridiculous or raise you up to your better self.

Finally, when it comes to happiness and fulfilment, donating time often does more than donating money, and gives you more joy. We consider our society so advanced and yet our world is beset with social, economic and environmental issues.

If you are reading this book then you are better off than the 775 million people in the world who cannot read. We shudder at the lack of sewers there were in the past, yet we pollute our planet at an exponential rate. We scorn at the inequality people once faced, yet remain ignorant of the harsh conditions millions work under to provide us with cheap consumables. Donating time to others or important causes connects us with a higher purpose, giving a more sustained version of joy compared to a new gadget. I encourage you to seek out those opportunities that make a difference in our communities and profession.

Everything You Think You Know Might be Nonsense

Information that you accept as fact could be shown to be a fallacy in the future. Consider that minds as bright as yours once thought the world to be flat or believed that trepanning (the practice of drilling holes in the skull) was the best treatment for migraines. The people of these times presented evidence that seemed to confirm without doubt that their beliefs were based on sound facts. Might chiropractic practice be scoffed at by future generations?

Chiropractic has faced scrutiny since its incarnation. Facing scrutiny for a perceived lack of evidence for unbelievable outcomes. The saving grace has been one undeniable fact; Chiropractic works. When insurance companies in the USA started to cover chiropractic care, it shifted the public perception of chiropractors to become back and neck pain specialists, thus research funding focused on validating chiropractic as a treatment modality. Due to the switch in research, the benefits of Chiropractic on overall health have not been fully explored.

The profession walks a tightrope, aiming to provide

evidence for its outcomes, while not limiting itself to being associated solely with back and neck pain. This balancing act has created a rift within the profession that has loosely grouped chiropractors into "mechanists" and "vitalists".

One camp pushes for validation as pain specialists and to gain the respect from other medical professionals while rejecting all chiropractic concepts and terminology that they consider to be "non-evidence based". The other camp stays true to the traditions of Chiropractic, pointing to the promising evidence gained to date and the weight of testimonies from thousands of people whose lives have been changed when it seemed like all other forms of care were ineffective.

The difficulties in producing evidence may soon change as it is conceivable that in the near future smart technology will provide an insight into the effects of chiropractic. An individual may have years of qualitative, unbiased data about their health logged, before coming to see the chiropractor of the future. The perceived benefits to sleep quality, heart rate variability, digestion, headache frequency or even back pain will be put to the test.

Your role in our collective future as a profession is to stay open to the possibilities of how chiropractic care may impact an individual's nervous system and overall health, while retaining the ability to critically think and discount ideas you once thought were fact. We can all contribute to research that deepens our understanding and realise that the perceived rift in the profession is counterproductive to overall growth.

Those within Chiropractic who invest energy in maintaining this divide, often overlook the fact that the people utilising our care do not consider our terminology or beliefs important, they come to us for the services we provide and the positive impact on their lives. I believe the range in approaches is a strength for our profession and we must focus on the fact that we all help our communities in individual ways.

You Are Going To Die And You Have No Idea When Or How

Perhaps one of the most difficult subjects to discuss openly, is death. Our brains are hardwired to imagine a life where we have a rosy end to our existence, surrounded by our loved ones, after a long happy life. Reality is often different and sometimes tragic; fatal accidents, protracted illnesses or a slow decline into dementia are not uncommon. While death is assured, the manner and timing of it are great unknowns.

In Mexican culture there are 3 types of death. The first death happens when you first realise the concept of your own mortality; that you will one day die. The second death is when you actually die and your life is celebrated by those you leave behind. The third death is when the last person who remembers what you did in your life passes away, meaning your life is forgotten and merges with the millions of unnamed ancestors we have all had and that have led us to being alive and where we are today. Many people endeavour to lead a life of significance so that their actions are remembered beyond their lifetime. As to whether or not we are creating the legacy we hoped for, we can acquire objectivity in assessing the extent to which we are on course to do so by asking the following questions:

· If you died tomorrow would you be happy with what you've achieved?
· If you knew you had 10 years left on this planet what would you do to make a positive impact on the world?

- If you have an answer to these questions what can you start to do now to make that positive impact happen?

The unseen enemy that prevents ambitious goals from being achieved lies within your own head. For millennia, our ancestors faced a struggle for survival, focused on immediate problems rather than planning for retirement. Our logical brain knows we should do what is best, but often our need for instant gratification wins out. That is why you may have a shelf full of books you have promised you will read one day, while you spend evenings absorbing hours of junk TV. If you truly want to attain those big goals in life then you must cultivate habits and systems that allow you to overcome your procrastinating brain to make the most of whatever time you have.

BJ Palmer's famous quote, "*We never know how far-reaching something we may think, say or do today will affect the lives of millions tomorrow*", sums up the sentiment that our daily actions can have a significant impact on a future we cannot even imagine. One person can achieve a lot in their lifetime, with persistent actions focused on their purpose. That person's purpose can grow so big that it continues to expand beyond their lifetime and creates a legacy, like the chiropractic profession.

Wisdom #10

Sarah Farrant DC

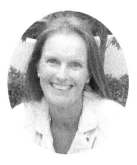

Sarah is the co-founder of Vital Wellbeing, a company dedicated to optimising the health of multiple generations by providing vital tools for generational change in health globally. This is done in 3 ways: direct services (Move), the Vital Foods line (Eat) and their online education (Think), all of which have led to her receiving numerous leadership awards and much media interest.

Sarah is an award winning, global selling, Amazon #1 author of 2 books, The Vital Truth and The Health Illusion which are sold in over 34 countries. Since the 1990's, Sarah and her husband have been global mentors to thousands of people, helping change many lives.

Trust the process

In 2001, I was pregnant for the first time. My husband Randall and I were living in Davenport, Iowa, three quarters of the way through our Palmer College programme. We had made connections with the Amish community, where we found our midwives. Midwives who at the time had been at the feet of home-birthing mothers over 2,000 times, with 25 sets of twins and only one stage-3 complication.

Twice a month on Saturday mornings, we used to drive through the blistering Illinois winter snow to their farm, to collectively converse with other couples about our pregnancies. We'd take food to share, sit on the floor and chat for hours.

When it came time for me to share one Saturday morning, I drew a huge breath, closed my eyes, plucked up some courage and blurted, "I don't trust my body to birth."

Tears welled in my eyes and my body started to shake as I continued to share how scared I was. I *did* trust myself to nurture and develop our child through pregnancy and I *did* trust myself in parenting, but I didn't trust my body to birth.

Several months went by and I created the opportunity to experience birth; a miscarriage of our twins at 14 weeks at home. During my miscarriage experience I kept saying over and over the 3 words our midwives had shared with me, *trust the process.* Even though I was studying Chiropractic and the innate intelligence of the human body, plus the associated trust that comes with that knowledge, my Achilles heel was I wasn't applying my knowledge. I loved our chiropractic philosophy classes and I understood what was being taught at an intellectual level, however up until this experience, I hadn't been living it fully.

By having the experience of a birth, through a miscarriage at home, with no intervention or post dilate and curate, I was able to develop an unwavering trust in myself and apply it to my life. Post the birth I got to experience my mind and my body going through an innate process of healing. It was like flicking on a switch. I went on to have three very beautiful and different home births. Anam was born with the Amish midwives in Davenport, Iowa, USA. Rui was born in Queensland, Australia with my husband and a chiropractic colleague, and no midwife present. Anais was also born at home in Queensland. Her birth was the ultimate experience of trust, as I knew she was breech. We had no midwife associated with her pregnancy but we did with her birth. Each experience gave me the opportunity to cement further into this process of trust.

Prior to bringing kids into the world, Randall and I were living a great life – working and travelling the world and eating in great restaurants for 11 years. When we decided to have kids, we also decided to be congruent in our education with them about health, the human body and its expression. We agreed we would start with making sure our actions and language matched our philosophy on health. We wanted to use words that would be empowering to our kids rather than confusing and fear driven.

In 2002, before the birth of our eldest, I was playing with words and created the word "health expression" to replace the more commonly used word, "sickness". I define health expression as 'a condition of expressing the whole you' where health means 'wholeness', express means 'to express,' and ion means 'a condition of'. You might use health expression in your house too and if you do, I'm honoured. It is used by chiropractors all over the world, by health professionals who have picked up on its uniqueness, and the general public too.

The origin of the word "sickness" stems from being ill, diseased, feeble, weak, deeply affected and troubled. I didn't want our kids to think of their body in that manner, I didn't want them to feel like something had to be fixed, nor feel the need go to someone to get something to take something away. I wanted them to live knowing that they had the potential to create and experience unlimited possibilities to change throughout their physical life time; not just in health but in all areas of their life. I wanted them to trust the process, their body and the genius that lives within; and live a different health and life paradigm.

Each of our kids, in their own unique way, have created

health expressions; these opportunities for themselves to change – physically, chemically and emotionally. They have created fevers, rashes, worms, self-confidence concerns, lice, diarrhoea, vomit, tears, abrasions, sprains, bumps and bruises, deep long-lasting coughs, turmoil, colds, headaches, concussions, bee and wasp stings, stress and friendship challenges.

We adjust our children every Friday morning and have done so since they were minutes old. Our point of difference to others is how we handle those challenges; the explicit trust we have, the conversations we have, the language we use, the actions we demonstrate, and the questions we ask, all of which make the difference in embracing a health expression or not. When our kids create these opportunities, they don't hear us saying "You caught this", "You got this", "This happened to you", "Poor you", "Here take this, it will make you feel better", "This will fix it", and so forth; all disempowering statements that would have you live life in and with fear.

When our kids have created a health expression either physically, chemically or emotionally, we have been the nurturers of *their* experience. We have provided an environment for them to express whatever needed to be expressed. We have trusted in their bodies to heal and grow. We have never offered them a medication – over the counter, prescribed or scheduled, nor have we ever taken them to a medical doctor, a naturopath or a homeopath. We have educated them about opportunity and the wisdom of the body. We have told them that the greatest gifts come 10 to 14 days following the creation of a health expression. We have got excited with them; we have celebrated their health expression.

In some cases, it is like flicking on a switch, you can see the physical growth, hear the language change and notice the emotional maturity. In other cases, it is more subtle, like a switch in the vegetables they eat or a change of a habit. We didn't say no or deny medications, but we said yes to trust, and as a result our experience of our kid's health challenges has been very different to most. By virtue of living in a different health paradigm, with its different values, language and actions, we have had a very different health experience; everything changes.

Just as we have the opportunity to see either sickness or a health expression, the same can be applied to the subluxation. Has the body got it wrong when getting a subluxation and therefore a person "needs" to go to someone (chiropractor) to get something (an adjustment) to take something away (fix it, remove it), so the sick person can become well? That's a rather mechanistic and allopathic approach to the subluxation. Or has the body created, through the subluxation, an evolutionary opportunity to change physically, chemically and emotionally, which is vitalistic and alternate in its approach? This latter approach to the subluxation, as with a health expression, engenders trust.

In 1999 I was honoured to be asked by Lori Leipold at Palmer College of Chiropractic to facilitate a philosophy discussion during Lyceum, between 4 of our great philosophers - Fred Barge, Reggie Gold, Victor Strang and David Koch. There were pre-set questions I had to ask. The audience was full to capacity at Palmer's Lyceum Hall. The stage was set.

Lori whispered to me backstage, "Sarah, you're up!" I quietly walked over to collect the clip board, "Would it be okay if I asked a question of my own?" I whispered back to her. "No, you can't go off brief," came the reply. "Oh, okay," I replied, with a disappointed tone.

I walked onto the stage and in front of thousands of people I began to ask these philosophy greats the pre-set questions. The audience was into it and the philosophers were on fire sharing some absolute gems of wisdom. I saw out the corner of my eye Lori, hidden behind the curtain backstage, rolling her hands indicating to me that I needed to wrap it up.

The clock was ticking and my internal voice kept saying over and over, "It's now or never Sarah." Time was called. I dug deep inside to pluck up as much courage as I could and halted the closing. "I have one more question for you all", I blurted. And then out it came, "Do you think subluxations can be of benefit for the evolution of mankind?"

I asked this question because up to that point our subluxation education had been mechanistic in its approach - it's bad and needs to be removed to help sick people get well. I wanted to flip that understanding on its head.

There was a deathly silence. You could hear a pin drop. And then the crowd in unison started chanting, 'Boo! Boo!" Some rose to their feet and started to fist pump the air with the echo of the booing. If food was allowed in the hall then I would have been fruit salad. Fred Barge stopped the booing and said, "I believe you are onto something." While looking at each of his colleagues he said, "I think there need to be some timely deaths so that the profession can advance forward." He passed away only a few years later.

As I left the stage and the auditorium, I had people chase after me saying, "How can a subluxation be beneficial?" And, "What's this evolution of mankind bullshit?" While I wasn't scared, I had certainly played my card and I still had a couple of years left of college! However, I was pleased that I had instigated a new conversation.

To wrap this all up, in order to get to the core of our trust we need to be able to break our own illusions that we carry about health and the subluxation, and ask different and refreshing questions. For me, a subluxation is an opportunity, just like a health expression; an opportunity to change physically, chemically and/or emotionally. The adjustment is not a quick fix; it is an opportunity to integrate one's life.

I believe a person creates a subluxation via their perceptions of their world and they see that perception simply as either good or bad. Either way, the perception alters a person's physiology via their nerve system and a unique set of signs and symptoms are created for that person to experience. A subluxation, just like a health expression, is the opportunity by which we can instigate change.

Trusting the process is paramount to seeing the benefit of its role in the evolution of our life. All things have their time, their place, their moment. As we learn more about the world we live in and the genius that lives within, we see glimpses of the illusions that have governed us and we see opportunities to change and evolve.

Kelly-Jane McLaughlin DC

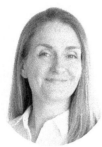

Kelly-Jane has run a busy, family-based practice in Reading, UK along with her husband Liam, for the past 10 years. She is also a devoted mum to 3 busy boys, all of whom are home-birthed, un-medicated and home educated.

An inspirational teacher, Kelly trains chiropractors across Europe in how to build family-based practices with a specific focus on caring for pregnant ladies. She is co-founder of Hayley and Kelly, a business running retreats for like-minded people which also has a growing online forum hosting international speakers in all areas of health and wellbeing.

Discovering what makes me TIC

I remember the first time I realised Chiropractic was so much more than I knew. You see, unlike most of the other students who started chiropractic college with me, I had never seen a chiropractor or been checked or adjusted before I started chiropractic school! I did not have a miracle story or really know what chiropractic was. I did not experience an adjustment until halfway through my first year at college. Still, something pulled me to chiropractic school to study, to be able to join this amazing profession.

That something was very different from what I originally thought. Then, 3 things happened in my second year of chiropractic school. These 3 things would forever change my understanding of what Chiropractic - and life - was. They would shape me to be able to work in the way I do and share the gift and magic of chiropracTIC with others.

The first "moment" occurred when I was invited as a guest to attend the first Chiropractic Essentials. I remember sitting in the audience and a chiropractor called Adrian Wenban was speaking on stage. He spoke about research and how it pertains to the chiropractic understanding of health and life. It was more advanced than anything I had ever heard. In among that information, he said this (and I apologise if the words are slightly different but this is how they stay in my memory), "The likelihood of life happening by chance is the same likelihood as a whirlwind blowing through your back yard and constructing a Boeing 747." He spoke about how life is not a series of random events and how health is not based on "luck".

He probably spoke for half an hour after that comment, but my mind had already exploded; how could I not have ever heard this before? If this was true (and every part of me knew it was, regardless of him giving us the statistics and research to explain and prove it was) then everything I had been taught and knew about life was not as I believed!

I went back to lectures and thought about this continuously. I had not heard this understanding of Chiropractic and life while at college, I was not being taught this. It started to make me question what I was learning. Was I being taught the truth about Chiropractic?

The second 'moment' was a few months later when Guy Riekeman DC came to speak at our college. Again, he spoke of so many interesting topics and was really motivating. I was enjoying his presentation but the words I remember most were centred around this question he asked us. He said: "Who here has taken antibiotics?" Of course, being a child of the 1980s/1990s,

I raised my hand. He then asked, "And those of you who have, who thinks they saved them and healed them?" Well of course, I raised my hand and agreed. What exactly was his question here? The final part of this speech would rock me for months!

He proceeded to tell us that the antibiotics did not actually heal us and that he had never given his children antibiotics. He started to talk about the body's ability to heal itself and introduced me to "innate intelligence". Well, by this stage I was now really cross! How could someone who seemed so clever be saying these things to us? I was riled and annoyed. It just could not be true! I left that presentation still mad that someone could know so much and so little at the same time. Wow, if only I knew.

Fast-forward to spring of that year and my third "moment" would occur. I was presented (by someone who had just been to a Koren seminar weekend) with a huge lever arch folder full of all sorts of information and the words, "You HAVE to read this! You will love it. This is amazing." When I opened the folder, on the first page was a poem called The Big Idea. The man who gave me that folder is now my husband and tears prick his eyes every time he reads the poem! I do not know if either of us knew at that time the significance of those words and how they would shape our lives now.

So, with this information, my mind being expanded, and eyes opened, I turned into a seminar junkie. I could not get enough information. I needed to know more about this brilliant "idea". I needed to learn more about what these things meant, and I needed to know more about Chiropractic, no one at college spoke of it, it was like a guarded secret. I wanted in on that secret, badly!

So, years went by, my knowledge and understanding grew

and I took my first real job with a fabulous couple in Carlisle. I read my contract from them and one of their terms was "to respect the innate intelligence of the practice". I called my Mum. These people are amazing, I want the job and know I will learn loads, but - what was this about? How very odd and strange. What were they talking about? Clearly, I had not opened my eyes as much as I thought. I signed it anyway; something made me buzz and by now I had learned that those feelings lead to great discoveries. My first 3 years in practice shaped me (I hear this a lot now about how important it is to choose your first job role carefully; it fast-tracks you to where you want to go). Christophe Vever DC taught me more about ChipraTIC, the power of the body and the importance of excellent communication skills in 3 months than I had learnt in my whole 5-year degree. Those skills are still vital today when it comes to my communication with everyone about ChiropracTIC.

After 10 years in practice, my husband and I started to coach with Sarah Farrant DC. Our life would take a 180 degree turn and finally, for me, all the pieces of this brilliant jigsaw were put into place. Now, not only did I understand ChiropracTIC but I could apply this throughout my whole life. After all, when you understand TIC you realise it could never be separate! It took years, the usual grumpiness (from me) and then the revelation. We had at the same time opened our practice together and spent a few years fine-tuning things to the way we wanted and we practised sharing the chiropractic story. Anyone who has worked in their own practice knows how brilliant and how very challenging it can be. I am not sure when it changed for me but somewhere along the way of driving a business forward, juggling life and acting out the motions, I had lost my

ChiropracTIC mojo. I did not realise this at all until I was given a very precious gift. I had a call from a dear friend whose baby had arrived very early. They were in hospital, in ICU, and asked me if I would come and check their new baby and help them. Without hesitation of course I said yes.

On the drive over, I started to question myself. What could I do to help? Why would I be able to contribute anything to them in this situation? It seemed almost fake to me to even agree to go, after all, so many others could help them better. Standing outside the security door to the ward, I waited for much longer than I needed to, questioning. I probably would still be standing there if a relative had not come out and met me. I was taken into the ward. Now, for anyone who has been on an ICU ward you will know that it is a crisis environment. It is frankly scary. That was the moment it hit me hard. This was not about me. This was about something way bigger than I could ever find the words to explain. This was about an intelligence that is in all of us, a reflection of the universal intelligence that connects us all. I was here to deliver a gift that would never come from me, but I had the privilege to ensure it could come through me. The baby was nestled at my friends' breast, not feeding but comforted all the same.

When I placed my hands onto the baby's atlas, for the first time her baby started to suck and to feed. They were told this would not be possible as the baby had been born too early. We knew. People will say that a wonderful thing occurred that day; a baby was able to feed and thrive. A wonderful thing did occur that day; I was reminded of the power of the gift we are given, of something far bigger and more vital than ourselves! On the shoulders of giants, we stand.

Wisdom #11

Stew Bittman DC

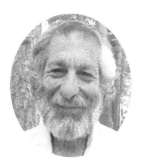 *Stew has travelled a long road in his 38 years in Chiropractic. Having initially struggled in practice, he discovered the chiropractic principle and began a journey of transformation to go on to own a high volume, vitalistic practice. Much of that time he travelled, taught and spoke alongside Jim Sigafoose, becoming one of the most inspiring speakers in the profession.*

As the creator of Chiropractic from the Heart workshops, Stew opens hearts through all that he does. He is an ordained interfaith minister and a published author. In 2009 he retired from practice and ministry but continues to coach, speak and lead workshops in Chiropractic.

The heart of Chiropractic

I embarked on my journey in Chiropractic nearly 40 years ago and the subsequent 4 decades seem like a blur. A beautiful, fulfilling, joyful blur. I sincerely appreciate the opportunity to write this chapter because it forces me to slow down the blur and reflect upon it. When I do, the years become a long collection of stories that have become the tapestry of my life. In this chapter I share some of my favourite stories because they illustrate the deepest truths about Chiropractic that I know - the ones that hold that tapestry together.

The stories in this chapter also demonstrate how truly unique Chiropractic is. For various reasons over the 125 years of its history, Chiropractic has portrayed itself as a variety of things with a variety of purposes and therefore public perception about it is unclear to this day.

For me, the list of things Chiropractic is NOT is considerably longer than the list of things it is.

If there is a prevalent public opinion about Chiropractic, it is that it's essentially a therapy for back pain, neck pain and headaches. There's no denying that Chiropractic can be incredibly helpful for those things; indeed, over the years I've seen those and a vast range of other symptoms and conditions get better under chiropractic care. Yet, Chiropractic is not a therapy for anything.

Chiropractic recognises and relies upon an inborn intelligence or organising principle within the body that under all circumstances is working to maintain balance and ease. The purpose of a chiropractic adjustment is simply to remove interference to the expression of that intelligence so that balance and ease can be restored. It differs from a therapy or treatment, therefore, because those things imply something done TO the body to directly deal with a symptom or condition.

With a chiropractic adjustment, the power for healing or change is already within the person being adjusted. With a therapy, the power has to lie within the practitioner or in the therapy itself. This obviously requires knowledge about both the problem and ways to bring things back more towards "normal." As a chiropractor, my focus was always on the former and that is undoubtedly why the most miraculous and memorable things that changed for people in my practice were things I didn't know anything about before they changed.

Faye came in for help with lower back pain after many years of waitressing. She embraced the chiropractic message and her care was helpful on many levels in her life, including for her back. One day she was in tears and told me she'd just visited her kidney specialist and was informed she didn't need to have dialysis treatments that had already been scheduled. Her kidneys had improved from 20% function to 90% in the past year with no change in her medical treatment. Faye said, "I never told you about my kidneys because I didn't think you could do anything about them." I replied, "You were right! But apparently the intelligence within you knew what to do about them."

Around that same time there was a gentleman in my practice who complained of shoulder pain and repeatedly asked me when it would feel better. Each time I replied with some version of, "I don't know, because I'm not adjusting you to make your shoulder feel better. I'm adjusting you to remove interference to the expression of life within you, so that the intelligence that took atoms from the environment and used them to create your body and that vigilantly maintains you in an incomprehensible state of balance and harmony can have free reign to do whatever it needs to do. That intelligence created your shoulder and re-creates your shoulder and undoubtedly knows how to recreate it more normally but there's really no way for me to know how long that will take or even IF it will happen. Perhaps there are more important priorities it needs to work on right now." My replies weren't always that long, but that was always the message.

This literally went on for 2 months, twice a week. I began to think he might be in the wrong place for his care. I checked in with him to see if something else in his life had improved but he hadn't noticed anything. Then, in the process of suggesting to him that he might seek care elsewhere, his 5-year-old daughter told me he had stopped beating her since he'd started getting adjusted.

If relief of shoulder pain had been the goal, then Chiropractic failed miserably. If I had known he was beating her, I wouldn't have had a single clue as to how to help him. Or her. Indeed, my legal responsibility at that point would have been to report him to the authorities. As it stands, there is no episode in my long years in Chiropractic that lends more evidence to its beauty nor its simplicity, its frequently dramatic positive impacts, or how it stands distinct from any therapy; except perhaps for my mission trip experiences in Panama, Costa Rica and the Dominican Republic.

On these trips, thousands of people received the gift of chiropractic care (on our third trip to Panama in 1998, 147 Chiropractors adjusted almost 400,000 people in 6 days). In most cases, the language barrier prevented us from finding out why folks had come to be adjusted or what might have been "wrong" with them. This was perfect, because chiropractic is much more concerned with what is "right" with people; the intelligence within them.

Of course, we'll never know what happened for all those people, but we do know that a little deaf girl had her hearing return after one adjustment on our first mission. We saw a young woman get out of her wheelchair for the first time in 12 years. We were told that children in institutions where we adjusted were smiling for the first time in their lives. Several people shared through interpreters that they had been contemplating suicide before getting adjusted. On our fourth mission to Panama, we were told by the mayor of Panama City that the crime rate there had gone down significantly after our third trip. Beyond what we witnessed and heard, we FELT the entire vibration of the country change on every mission.

I don't know of any therapy that can accomplish all that. I do know that what we accomplished on these trips was not due to our personalities or our skills or our words. It was due to our ability to fully open our hearts and serve the purest version of Chiropractic that we'd ever expressed to that point. We were able to keep all our attachments and expectations out of the way, and the power that was already within the folks we adjusted poured forth undimmed.

After my mission trip experiences, my life's purpose became about continuing to open my heart so both my practice folks and I could experience that same magic back at home. Our practice got a bit closer to that every day. From ushering babies into the world, to being midwives for elderly folks making their final transition. In helping all the folks in between to navigate their lives more fully connected to their highest vision, our practice became a centre of light and hope.

As I write this, the world is reeling over Covid-19 and chiropractor centres are some of the only places of certainty, light and hope available to people. So, I continue to hold a vision of certainty, light and hope catching fire; a world in which everyone knows the value of chiropractic principles and receives chiropractic care, and therefore a world in which everyone is valued and everyone, including the planet, thrives.

So, what exactly is Chiropractic? After all these years and all these stories, I find it harder than ever to pigeonhole it into any pre-existing category.

Chiropractic care is wonderful for one's health and wellbeing, but it isn't just healthcare. Chiropractic is a way of life that offers hope, certainty and peace of mind, but it isn't just a philosophy or belief system. Chiropractic is unique because it espouses a set of timeless, universal principles AND offers a practice and an art that can powerfully bring those principles to life. I have discovered it takes both to make the greatest positive impact on people's lives and on the world.

The world could certainly use a huge dose of both right now.

I left the chiropractic profession for 12 years to pursue ministry and lead a non-denominational spiritual centre here in Lake Tahoe, California. The principles of the spiritual movement I was involved in are essentially the same as Chiropractic's and I had the advantage of "preaching to the choir" in that all the congregants already believed in those principles. Yet right away my wife and I observed that folks in our congregation were not making the huge changes in their lives that we had observed in our chiropractic practice. It just didn't have the same impact without the adjustments.

What is Chiropractic? If you take the principles of quantum science and all the spiritual traditions throughout the ages, distill them down to their most practical elements and then add a beautiful art form, involving the laying on of hands, to bring those elements into living expression, you end up with Chiropractic.

After 40 years of miraculous stories, I can clearly see they are all about hearts opening. Chiropractic adjustments, especially when delivered with love and with no attachment to a specific outcome (other than the certainty of some positive result), reconnect people to everything that is good, beautiful and true about them and within them. Chiropractic adjustments re-awaken folks to their deepest values, their highest potential, and the biggest, truest version of themselves.

Chiropractic adjustments reunite folks with their dreams and because of that, I've led a dream life. No words could ever describe the gratitude I feel every day for my beloved profession.

Heidi Brown DC

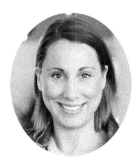

Despite building a thriving wellbeing practice with great client retention, chiropractor and business owner Heidi struggled with self-confidence, never feeling good enough. Over the years she found it essential to do deep inner work, which has allowed her to transform her self-worth and discover her gift and passion for helping others to do the same.

Heidi's focus is now mostly on coaching and running retreats, where she can gently challenge you to go deep within yourself and identify your blocks, so you can ultimately express more of yourself and uncover more of your gift.

Learning to trust yourself

I was lucky enough to experience Chiropractic from a young age. My mum met a really charismatic chiropractor, Steve, at my primary school playground, and from that one conversation my whole family started care. Of course, I didn't think much of it at the time. It was just something I did. When it came to choosing my career, chiropractic wasn't even on my radar. I liked biology, and helping people, so counselling and physio were top of my list. I think the reason chiropractic wasn't even a consideration is because my whole family viewed Steve as a miracle worker, a healer. He was larger than life. So bold, unconventional, certain. It never even crossed my mind that it was a profession that others could do, and certainly not me. I was nothing like him.

Then through a bizarre twist of circumstances (I know, I know, Chiropractic chooses you) I ended up doing work experience with Steve. I got to see so many amazing things that week, but I'm embarrassed to admit that that wasn't what did it. It was observing another associate, who seemed much more 'human', conventional, quiet; more like me. Yet she was beautiful, chic and respected. She seemed really comfortable in her own skin, which is what I was desperate for. It was the promise of that, rather than the Chiropractic itself, which put me on the path to chiropractic college.

I came out of university feeling unprepared for what was ahead. I wasn't confident in my adjusting skills and I was confused between the vitalistic model I had grown up with, versus the musculoskeletal model I'd been taught at university. I was deeply convinced about the importance of chiropractic care for everyone, but I lacked the ability and confidence to communicate this to my clients. I quickly realised that the effortless fulfilment I'd been expecting wasn't going to come. Graduation hadn't given me the personality transplant I was hoping for, and I hadn't magically become as talented and confident as Steve. He was still up high up on a pedestal and I was falling short. I felt I was failing in every way. I was lost.

I went on so many technique seminars in those first few

years, desperate to learn more so that I would start to feel confident in what I was doing. All of it helped, a bit. I developed a wide range of techniques I could use, and even though I didn't feel I had mastered any of them, I certainly grew in my capabilities and confidence. However, I was really missing my grounding in chiropractic philosophy. Everything I was doing felt a bit hollow.

Eventually I found my tribe. People who were talking about Chiropractic the way I knew it; vitalistic, passionate, certain. It felt like I was coming home. The speakers I heard on stage had an infectious enthusiasm for Chiropractic, and a deep knowledge of body and soul. They seemed like giants, miracle workers, philosophers. They would talk about chiropractic adjustment with such reverence. The miracles they were getting, the amount of people they were helping, their busy, successful practices, the money they were earning; it was hugely inspiring.

But only to a point.

While I loved hearing their stories and successes, very quickly that inspiration turned into a deep self-judgement. Why wasn't I getting miracles with every single client? I didn't leave my day feeling more energised than when I started. I wasn't seeing the same numbers they did. I couldn't earn as much. I wasn't practising open plan, which seemed to mean I wasn't vitalistic enough. The list of things I could reprimand myself for seemed endless. All that inspiration, rather than motivating me to build the practice of my dreams, became yet another reason why I wasn't good enough. An excuse to beat myself up. To feel less than. I had huge respect for chiropractic and vitalistic principles, I just didn't feel that I was good enough to deliver them.

The Wisdom of 33

That led me to thinking, as I'd start adjusting a client, doing that first leg-length check, "Surely if this client was seeing someone else, they would have had a miracle by now, their posture would be perfect, they would have made more lifestyle changes, or brought their whole family in for care, or referred more people to me." Those thoughts swirled around my head all day. I had created a prison for myself.

I felt exhausted, burnt out.

I kept going to seminars, desperate to find the silver bullet to make everything ok. That perfect technique to cure everyone. The one communication strategy that worked every time. That insight into myself that would fix what must be broken inside me. I couldn't understand why I didn't feel confident in who I was, why I wasn't enjoying practice. But it was to no avail. At each seminar I would love it, feel inspired, but within a few hours I would have created a sore throat, swollen glands - my tell-tale sign of "I'm not good enough", and the experience would just reinforce that I was less than.

I eventually found some personal development work that was unlike anything I had done before. During a week-long retreat in Ireland, I uncovered a lot of the things that were holding me back. I was able to find understanding around why I was the way I was, and to feel some compassion for myself. I left that week feeling like I mattered, for the first time in my adult life. I had value. I was enough. Everything felt lighter, easier. The internal shift was immense. From the outside, barely visible, but on the inside, everything was different.

That deep inner work enabled me to appreciate the practice I had created. Rather than viewing everything through the automatic lens of failure and other people's goals, I could enjoy it based on what I wanted and valued. I quickly realised that by my standards, I actually did have a thriving practice. Clients were coming to get checked regularly, year after year. They felt cared for and nurtured by me and my team. I got to appreciate the beauty of the space I was able to hold for them. There would often be tears, as clients felt truly seen and heard, maybe for the first time in a long while. I had a waiting list for new patients and at various stages of practice, for adjustments too. I had a Patient Visit Average (PVA) in the hundreds.

It was then that I realised that for me, Chiropractic is so much more than the individual skill of an adjustment, or the scientific knowledge we have. I had always been frustrated that clients didn't understand all the neurology behind what we were doing. They didn't get as excited as I was about the changes we were making to their brain. However, as I let go of this, I started to appreciate that it was the whole experience of how they felt in themselves during and after their visit that mattered so much more. It was this that kept them wanting to come back year after year. Finally, that was a good enough reason for me.

The other huge shift I made after that retreat was in readjusting my expectations of clients. I've been consumed by Chiropractic and its philosophy for years, and there are still areas where I come unstuck. I realised that it was unrealistic of me to expect people to "get it" at their report of findings and completely change their life. I realised that where I had felt broken myself, I had unknowingly transmitted that into how I practiced. I would talk about Chiropractic as a way to help people achieve their optimum potential, whatever that was for them. Really, deep down, I viewed Chiropractic as something that could fix everything. While I didn't feel whole and complete as a person, and I still needed fixing myself, that was what I tried to do for everyone else too. I felt deeply disappointed if any aspect of someone's health, physical, chemical or emotional, wasn't perfect. My mission to fix my clients was exhausting, and an impossible burden to bear.

As soon as I had built up my own self-worth, that expectation on myself and my clients shifted. It was liberating. Everything about practice became more effortless, more fun. It didn't drain me in the same way. I still worked very hard on showing up as the best me, but I released the pressure and expectations I put on my clients to transform.

As I look back on my chiropractic journey, I feel some sadness that I didn't figure this out sooner. I'm struck by how different it could have been. All those years of not trusting myself, and looking to others to define success for me. It feels so ironic that once I improved my own self-worth, and became congruent with what mattered to me, there was actually very little in my practice that I wanted to change. All those years where I'd felt miserable, the joy was right in front of me; I was living it each day, if I'd just given myself permission to experience it.

Being a very sensitive soul, I feel things more deeply than most. It's a great gift for my coaching work, but it means my awareness of what isn't quite right in my day-to-day life is intensified. My hope is that for many, this story will seem far more dramatic than theirs. I hope you will find comfort that you are not alone in feeling the way you do. My other wish is for those who are pushing and pushing for success and who are achieving what they thought they wanted but maybe are surprised that it doesn't come with the fulfilment they were expecting and it doesn't make them as happy as they wanted. Take a moment to reflect on why that might be. Look at whose goals you are trying to reach.

One of Chiropractic's most important philosophies to me is that we are healing and living life from the inside out. We all talk about it a lot, but the more I coach people, the more I witness that so many of us are deferring to others, someone or something outside our self, to define our success, and even our happiness. We spend our lives trying to live up to other people's expectations of us, or other people's goals. Whether it's living up to what we interpret that our parents wanted for us, or a predetermined definition of external success from speakers, Facebook, Instagram; it drains the life and enjoyment out of all we do, weakening our immune systems, our resilience. It's literally killing us in some cases.

Once you can appreciate who you are, your lightness and your darkness, your beauty and your flaws, you will be able to tune into what Chiropractic, or fulfilment, or a great life is for you. Your goals become a place that you come from, rather than something you are chasing. You are able to trust yourself, your innate, your own wisdom. You can become grounded and aligned with who you are, how you want to show up in this world. That is what makes all the difference.

Wisdom #12

Liz Anderson-Peacock BSc, DC

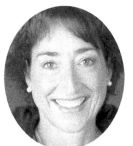

Liz is a curious soul. Described as insightful and in awe of the human spirit, she is a speaker, award-winning chiropractor and coach. She has contributed to clinical practice guidelines, peer reviewed papers, and supports many groups and associations.

Happily married and a grandmother of 5, she enjoys time spent in nature, water sports and painting, while still seeing patients after 34 years of being in practice. In 2017, she became a below-knee amputee but continues with all the things she did (and more) prior to her amputation with an even greater zest and reverence for life.

How has Awareness, Curiosity and Reverence impacted my practice life?

"Every day you make a difference of some sort and you have a choice as to what kind of difference you are going to make." - Dr. Jane Goodall

I will preface with a perspective that counters the predominant prevailing notion that the universe is inanimate and unintelligent. This perspective, while creating many discoveries, also has flaws. We have taken our planet, its life and interconnected systems, choosing to dissect and use as we deem fit, irrespective of the impact in doing so. In reducing ourselves to parts and unconnected silos we gain great information, yet with our compartmentalised lens how often do we forget that the parts interrelate?

Do we perhaps have an incomplete perspective causing us to miss solutions by asking different questions? Have we lost touch with what our body or our environment is telling us, only to give our power away to another? Is the body simply a machine to be used without respect for what we are doing to it? To be rebuilt and fixed before we carry on in the same way? Many times, I would say yes and I have done that. Does the body exhibit within it a living intelligence that holds all the known and yet unknown secrets enabling it to know how to reorganise, rebuild and heal itself given the right conditions? Yes, and I am a recipient of that too.

What order of magnitude would be required to get all things right such that our life exists? Or our universe for that matter?

Is there an intelligence working behind the scenes from a non-physical realm? If we exist within a field of information that is without form or material, that exists as vibration or frequency - wave form, can we tap into this vibrational consciousness? How is this even relevant in practice? I am asking you to improve your level of awareness of both the material - the body - and the immaterial.

Often patients say, "Put me back to where I was, doc!"

I sometimes answer, "Was that place really good in the first place? Or would a new place be even better?" It generates a great discussion.

Awareness is crucial in practice, and in life for that matter. One hears of situational awareness - being aware of what is occurring in the external environment outside us. It may signal danger or security. We also have internal awareness in our body providing messages like hunger, fatigue, thirst, etc; called interoception. Plus, we have emotions. Any which way we need to be "present" to notice, then interpret its meaning.

Have you been in another's company as the recipient of a singularly focused moment, where you lose track of time? A moment that feels like forever? Can we open our focus to be more aware of energy and vibration beyond our senses? I am sure you have experienced this with someone who is totally present with you. You momentarily feel like the centre of the world. Noticed. Significant. Seen. There is a loss of self, with an intangible connection.

Clinical practice is about noticing what's occurring, interpreting what it means, responding to information, deciding on a direction, implementing a plan, and observing an outcome. This requires accumulated knowledge, practical experience and constant reflection in concert with the patient.

Noticing requires paying attention, so as to gather data and this comes in tangible form through observation via our senses, assessments, tests, perhaps pattern recognition, and non-tangibly, through hunches and intuition. If we are not completely focused or present in the moment, we may miss a nuance that helps solve the puzzle. Opportunities arise throughout the day and we do not want to be too distracted or occupied to miss when or how they show up.

Awareness can come to us in the form of internal feedback. A gut feeling. A sixth sense. Something that causes us to re-evaluate. Perhaps it causes us to pause once more before we act.

Even if the initial path is unclear, when we pay attention to gathered information or evidence as we move to a new point in time, new information gathered provides feedback as to whether we are on the right path or need to add or delete something or pivot in another direction.

How does one get better at paying attention? It starts with oneself of course. My experience to date has been to master my basic knowledge, then to discipline myself to be more present in the moment. It requires me to be conscious rather than operate on autopilot. I have found I am getting better at picking up on clues when I am running an old programme. It shows up as being more distracted, more reactive and feels as though I am off course. I feel less internal ease and a huge red flag for me is when I try to control my environment. As I continue to be more aware of these behaviours, I am getting better at stopping, bringing my awareness to my chest through my breath and opening my heart until I feel reset. Like many things, it gets easier with conscious practise.

What I have experienced is that when I pay attention in the present moment, much more insight is gained. It is about having no agenda except having a singular focus right now. Tuning into the energy of the person. Not easy unless one practices. Probably like you, the mind goes to ruminating about past events or future thoughts that take up mental real estate. Life does not occur in the past and the future is yet unwritten. Life does occur in the here and now - the present. For me it is imperative to consciously bring my attention into the moment.

How does one achieve awareness? For me it requires quieting the active mind from analytical thinking. Calming the beta brain. Opening one's awareness to vibration or frequency; the non-tangible. Feeling the energy around, we then go into the "nothingness". This can be done through our breath, focusing on opening our heart.

Meditating. Getting lost in the moment, losing track of time without forcing, pushing, wanting or controlling. It requires surrendering, as in letting go and being open to receiving information in new ways. It takes practice and, in my mind, this is a noble endeavour because it adds another dimension to our care, in addition to using our other skills.

How often have you been with someone when they've been focused elsewhere? It doesn't feel good. They just weren't present.

I would encourage the discipline of exercises that support presence of mind and opening the heart. Perhaps it may sound crazy but when I have done this, there are times I feel like a vessel or I tap into a stream of consciousness where I am more connected, see patterns or all of a sudden questions/answers pop into my head that are the key that fit the lock of the problem before me.

Also helpful for presence and awareness, is keeping an open mind. Being flexible and available to receive information however it comes. With 5 grandchildren I am constantly reminded of their insatiable curiosity and their ability to question and learn. When applied to clinical care I believe we must be curious to learn new knowledge. We must be curious to question ourselves and others. We must want to problem solve. And we need to be curious to understand the patient's perspective. Their concerns, needs, wants, and values. We want to partner with the patient on a journey. Curiosity means staying flexible when it comes to dealing with a challenge, as there is often more than one way to solve a problem. We can use tried and tested ways, but if that doesn't work, we must think outside the box, if there is such a thing.

The value of a curious mindset is to consider possibilities and remaining teachable through active listening, observing and compassionately questioning others we may experience a different perspective that may very well fill gaps in our understanding and stimulate insight. As a result we may connect better with others.

My life has been governed both by a physical experience through my senses and this non-tangible awareness of something far greater than I.

This brings me to my third point. Reverence.

The potential buried within each of us is overwhelmingly beautiful. There is organisation in how the body creates and destroys itself, only to rebuild itself over and over again until our life cycle is done. In witnessing births and deaths there are moments of awe and grace as life begins, then comes full circle as it transitions and ends our human form. Reverence is so much more than compassion and kindness.

Reverence is deep respect for just how remarkable we are in our many forms, sizes, beliefs and colours.

Writer and speaker Wayne Dyer said, "*We are each a cell in the body of humanity.*" I would add that, "*Humanity is only as healthy as its weakest cell.*"

Reverence reminds me to see the potential buried within. When we see a caterpillar for the first time, we have no idea that it experiences metamorphosis to become a butterfly. What if we saw each other as emerging butterflies? Would we connect differently? How would we honour each other?

In seeing the potential within, the focus shifts from what's wrong and needs fixing, thus bringing them back to "normal", to helping them see the possibility and potential of a preferred future for themselves. Then we can work with strategies to move in that direction. Yes, there may be many obstacles. Yes, it requires commitment.

In the 1990s, I met Bernie Segal MD, a paediatric oncologist and author of Love, Medicine and Miracles. I remember his words on, "seeing the person who has the disease, not the disease who has the person."

Appreciate the beauty of this innate intelligence existing within our body. Have reverence that we are in a cycle of life with limitations to our physical form. Yet there exists the possibility to be so much more.

I learned this when, prior to my below-knee amputation, I was meditating and I experienced an indescribable wholeness with a deep loving connection and a message came to be that I am so much more than a body part. Minus part of my leg now, I couldn't agree more.

So, I will leave you with four questions:

What is your preferred future and how do you want to feel in it?

What might get in the way that you need to deal with in order to achieve this preferred future?

What is important to dedicate your resources to in order to achieve your preferred future?

If you applied this to health, vitality and wholeness what would be your first step?

Be present – see what happens.

Keltie Warren DC

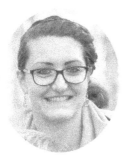

Dr Keltie Warren is extremely passionate about helping others reach their maximum potential. She is the owner of Warren's Chiropractic Café of Life, in Coldbrook, Nova Scotia. She has spent many years post-graduation learning about the brain and neurology and how to test optimal function in both.

She brings passion when she is speaking and mentoring. As a dedicated wife and mother of 3 beautiful children she fully understands the challenge of maintaining a healthy lifestyle while working in a busy world. She has developed peak strategies to be successful in both the office and life, and loves helping others discover the same.

Perspective: is what I'm telling myself true?

I sat down this morning to think about what I wanted to write for a chapter in a book about Chiropractic. There are so many options and so much in my mind that I feel I could write 20 books, but when it comes to actually putting my thoughts down on paper, it's paralysing.

My mind works a million miles a minute, going in a million different directions and then, self-doubt creeps in. Why you? Why would someone want to hear what you have to say? What value could you bring to the table? I can remember hearing as a child, "Kids' opinions don't matter, you're just a kid". But as a child it doesn't register as, "a child's opinion doesn't matter", it registers as "YOUR opinion doesn't matter, because it isn't of any value".

If you hear that message repeated often enough as a child, when you become an adult you may maintain the belief that you do not have anything of value to say. My parents didn't think what I said as a child was of any value, so why would someone want to pay for what I have to say now as an adult? But thanks to years of associating with the right people, instead of cowering to those thoughts and feelings of self-doubt and replying to the publisher with "you've picked the wrong person", I've learned to analyse those thoughts and feelings and question them. Why do I feel that way about myself? Who taught me that I was a lesser person and not worthy of speaking my truth? So, then it dawned on me and I decided that I would write about the importance of getting some perspective.

Before I get into discussing how we get perspective, I want to provide another example of an important issue that many adults struggle with. In addition to having self-limiting beliefs about the value of their opinions, many adults doubt their worthiness when it comes to having money. Anyone who has experienced their parents getting divorced, like I did, most likely understands how child support works. But if you have a father who repeatedly tells you as a child that you don't deserve the money he has to pay as child support, that can result in self-doubt as an adult regarding your worthiness of having any money. What my father may have meant was, "You're too young to decide how the money I provide is spent" (in my case my mother always gave me the money once I turned 18), but at the time it may have come across as, "You're not worthy of the money I provide".

Combine these 2 examples, and perhaps others, of self-value diluting messaging received as a child, and you have the perfect recipe for an adult who believes they have no valuable opinion to offer and they aren't worthy of being paid any money on whatever they produce. Imagine the effects of these beliefs on the adult who decides, like many chiropractors, to become an entrepreneur. This indeed would make for a very unsuccessful path.

How much of the world has these or similar issues to work through? Everyone. In some way or form we have all been conditioned by our past. The question is, "How does that conditioning present in the now?" I did a fun exercise with my 5-year-old this morning and asked her what do you think everyone should know about Chiropractic? Her answer: that you should get adjusted and it makes your body healthier, your body is always healthier after getting checked (and adjusted) multiple times, and your body should be healthy until you get checked again. I then asked her who she thinks should get adjusted and her eyes light up like a Christmas tree and she exclaimed "EVERYBODY!" So simple.

She gets it, or better yet she has been exposed to a positive idea for so long, it has become her own view. So, what we are exposed to becomes our reality and our understanding of the world. When we hold a view on the world and what it has to offer us, we have to ask where did that view come from and is it what we want to hold onto? Is that view serving us for our greater good? Until you learn to ask the questions of where a belief came from, you're most likely not going to be able to change and do any different.

I believe that is what's so powerful about Chiropractic, the effect the chiropractic adjustment has on our brain to make us able to evaluate and think differently. It opens our eyes to be able to better evaluate not only our current situation but past situations as well. It's only recently that I was able to look back and break an old thinking pattern about my past. I failed my first year of university. That's right, a GPA of 1.4. I had to redo almost every one of my classes. I felt massive shame around this. I believed I was stupid and lazy.

I've hidden that for years. Looking back, the month before heading into my first year of university I had a major horse-riding accident. I had a horse fall on top of me. I broke my thumb and the impact was so great I split my helmet and leather riding boot in two. That's a major impact, and because I was on my way to university, I stopped seeing my chiropractor (not a good excuse, but hey, I was 18). Then 8 months later I had even more severe concussion (the first one was undiagnosed, but looking back if you hit your head hard enough to split a riding helmet you probably have a concussion). I was tackled head-first into hockey boards while playing indoor rugby. I was walking and talking after the incident, but I have a one-to-two-hour window that I have zero memory of and have been told that I kept repeating the same question over and over again. So, was I stupid and lazy? Looking back, not at all! I had major head trauma that my body was trying to heal from. I'm so thankful that I later suffered a major hip issue that put me back into a chiropractic office, when I was in my third year of university.

Because of that first year of university, I thought I wasn't smart enough to be a chiropractor so I decided I was going to change my path and be a physiotherapist instead (to my physiotherapist colleagues and friends, please don't be insulted, I was under the impression that a physiotherapist was similar to a chiropractor, but the difference was that the former required a master's degree while the later required a doctor's degree. And I was of the belief I wasn't smart enough to be a doctor). I told my story to my chiropractor with shame and he flat out told me to smarten up, get back to class, get my grades up, and get to chiropractic school.

Thankfully, that was the pattern interruption that got me back on track. It was not just the words that he spoke, but the continued adjustments that allowed me to think more clearly and process information differently. If you have a self-belief, don't just accept it, question it. Where did it come from? Who told you? Why did they tell you? What was their experience? Were they doing their best?

Because of the repeated messaging I received in my childhood, I held the belief that I was either lazy or not smart enough to be in university and should drop out and not waste any more money. Where would I be now if I had accepted that version of myself without ever questioning it? My father asked me in my first year of being an undergraduate if I thought I was smart enough to do it. Thankfully, due to our rocky past, I often did things to prove him wrong or just out of spite.

Now I look back and realise his parenting was a repeated pattern and that in fact he was easier on me than his parents had been on him and that now it's my job to break the cycle completely. Instead of being angry with my past I digest all aspects with questions, rather than judgement. And as I sit writing this today, maybe my father wasn't insinuating I was stupid, he may simply have been asking can I do it?

Perspective is so powerful. I encourage everyone to stop when thinking about a past situation and simply ask questions. When you can do that, it's incredibly liberating. You can finally move past negative, ingrained patterns, behaviours, and self-limiting beliefs and see them for what they truly are; someone else's creations. Though, we can't completely absolve ourselves from all responsibility.

If you are a chiropractor, apply this understanding to the people who walk through your door for care. As chiropractors, we have something we want them to understand, but often we miss the boat because we don't know where they are originally coming from. Have they been taught that the body is brilliant and has an amazing ability to heal if it's given what it needs: no interference? Or have they been brainwashed into believing that they are weak and need the almighty MD to save them with a pill? When you realise that you have some de-conditioning to do, you lose the frustration and just get to work.

I truly believe the success of the chiropractic profession does not lie in how well we adjust (although that is valuable because we have to ensure we are producing what we say we do: a change through a specific adjustment). I believe it lies in our ability to change people's perspectives and belief systems. Once we can tap into their ability to think rationally, they will start to understand Chiropractic for what it is. Until we can do that, they may come to see us, but they will continue to default to their MD as the Holy Grail of health, and follow what they say, instead of seeing it for what it truly is: sick care that is necessary for emergencies only.

Wisdom #13

Pam Jarboe DC

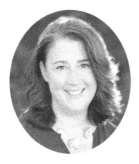

Dr Pam Jarboe practices Chiropractic in Acton, Massachusetts. Her career blossomed in 1986 when as a CA she travelled into Harlem, New York, with her chiropractor. He adjusted children who were drug addicted, some born with HIV who were abandoned as babies. Pam witnessed many transformations as they received their adjustments.

With less disease, less trauma, they stopped hiding under the beds, being terrified to be touched, to jumping into her arms. Inspired by the these and many other changes, especially in children, she graduated from Life Chiropractic University in 1995.

Dr Pam specialises in extraordinarily gentle chiropractic care. Her practices have always provided excellent care to people of all ages and health challenges. Dr Pam serves as a board member for several chiropractic organisations and is an international speaker for the profession. Her proudest contributions though, are her two sons, Jackson and Max.

"Alivening"

I sat across from a new 17-year-old patient in my office and took in the overall picture of him. He was contorted in a chair so that his left shoulder pressed against the back and his hips barely touched the chair. He was lethargic, had a black eye and his right arm was broken. His mom had called me late the night before, crying hysterically, telling me that her son had been involved with drugs and that it had gone very badly. He was hiding at a friend's house. He could not stay at home or "they" would find him. He owed them money and they had come to "encourage" payment. The woman was terrified. I had agreed to see him first thing in the morning and here we were. He had several broken ribs, a swollen eye, broken arm and was in tremendous pain. As we went through the history, he answered all my questions factually. He seemed nonplussed at his current situation. His mom knew the value of helping him to recover by increasing his neural integrity. He couldn't have cared less.

He was unable to write so I asked him about his personal history and at the end I asked how he would rate himself in the areas of physical health, mental health and overall quality of life. When I asked him about his self-assessments in the three categories mentioned above, he lit up. He rated himself as very healthy physically and mentally and when I asked about his quality of life, he enthusiastically added that he LOVED his life.

I have listened to people routinely minimise and distort their self-assessment for 25 years. But I was stunned at this level of contradiction. I fervently prayed that my face would not reveal my emotions and focused on typing. I continued to do the exam to the best of my ability and offered my care over the coming weeks. He was smuggled off to rehab and at this writing many years later, his mom reports that he is clean, sober and doing really well. His voice still reverberates around in my head as I contemplate how challenging it is sometimes to speak to patients about life.

This man-child highly valued numbness. His orientation towards numbness allowed him to rate his life as ROCKIN! If your goal is to be numb, living in the druggy world is the way to crush your life goals. This often catches chiropractors off guard. Chiropractors love life and want to be able to express more and more of it. They want to enhance the power of life through reducing blockages in the spine and through the chiropractic lifestyle. Their highest goal is to unite woman the physical with woman the spiritual. For them, numbness can feel like a crime. Chiropractors always want to dine at a Vegas-style buffet of life, while these civilians come in and scramble for crumbs off the table of life.

Much of the population we are working with are kindergarteners when it comes to consciousness. But we forget sometimes and try to speak to these kindergarteners as if they are in graduate school. My new patient exemplified this, clinging to the lowest rung of the ladder of consciousness. I could have spent an hour lecturing on health and wellbeing, vitality, protein shakes, stretching, breathwork, tree hugging, sagging, essential oils, colonic irrigation, ear candling and all the other things that seem so normal in the chiropractic lifestyle. The kindergartener in front of me who had convinced himself that his broken-rib-and-blackened-eye-world was perfect, would not have listened. I could have decided that he was a lost case, not my ideal client and dismissed him in my head, thinking, "NEXT". But I did not.

I did my job. I offered him specific, appropriate and effective chiropractic adjustments. And the power of life that moved through him allowed him to change. Not my lecturing, or all my righteous knowledge. In the few short weeks that I cared for him, I saw his muscular tension reduce, the intervertebral lack of motion increased, his respiration improved dramatically.

He commented on how amazing he felt after his adjustments. I explained that he had an innate pharmaceutical company within him. I explained that the nervous system influences the biochemistry of the body and that was why he felt so light and easy afterwards. He began to sleep more deeply and began to heal. What he needed from his brief experience with me, in my opinion, was to graduate out of numbness. The visceral experience of ease in his body that chiropractic adjustments offered, allowed him to go to his next step on human development, rehab.

Another time, a woman in her early 70s came in for a new patient appointment. She had a tremendous pain in her neck. Her history form included some benign physical history and most of the rest of the form had a line slashed through it to indicate it was not important. I had a "spidey" sense that there was much more going on here but I waited and continued the appointment as if that were true. I did a thorough examination on her, made recommendations and in the coming weeks, she started to receive successive adjustments. She had a reversed cervical curve and her musculature throughout the area was rigid. The individual vertebrae in her neck did not move. After a few weeks, some deep changes were happening.

But soon after, she came in and it was as if all the original parameters had returned. Her spine had gone backwards in progress. Before I adjusted her, I asked her to sit up. I asked her if anything was different in her life, because her spine seemed so different that day. She revealed that her son had been shot a few years ago, by a cheating spouse's boyfriend. Her son died and the daughter-in-law stopped all communication. So, she had lost her son and two grandchildren in one day, several years before. And on this particular day she was with me, there was a hearing to convict the daughter-in-law's boyfriend. She related this in a matter-of-fact way. Her body was visibly stiff as she shared, and I perceived that she was breathing very shallowly. I could see from her face that she did not want to talk about it. Or perhaps she did not know how. There was a part of me that wanted to rush to make it better. Fix it. Solve it. Stop It. And a part of me that desperately wanted to say The. Right. Thing. But the wisest part of me knew that in certain moments, the greatest gift we can give someone is our own courage to bear certain news. And share it. Even if for a moment.

So, I gently placed my hand on her shoulder, looked softly into her eyes and said, "I am so sorry." And then I was quiet. And I was with her. Truly. And she felt it. What I believe is that she knew that I was allowing myself to suffer even a minute fraction of what she had experienced. And she broke down sobbing. I mean, some of the most wretched grieving sounds I have ever heard. It lasted 5 minutes. But I stayed with her, hand gently on her shoulder. Not trying to do anything other than be with her. And allow this expression. She lifted her head at one point, took a deep breath and looked into my eyes. I met her gaze softly. She squeezed my hand on her shoulder and let me know she had not cried about it before. I handed her a tissue because so often in these moments, words fail. I held her shoulder for another moment and then said gently, "I am guessing that your body needed that so I am glad you were able to. Is it ok if I check your spine now?" Before I adjusted her, I noticed how much more pliable the tissue in her neck was, compared to earlier. Her whole body appeared to have so much more ease and breath.

I adjusted her that day and for many years after. I held in my mind the lyrics to *So Many Blessings by Steven Walters* which go, *"I don't want to take your pain away, I know that is your ticket home."*

So often as chiropractors we are trying to take away suffering and pain. We want to FixItStopItSolveIt. Sometimes we want that because we love people. Sometimes we want it so that we can FINALLY get recognition for how amazing we are. Or how amazing our product is. We think we are doing a good job if and when we fix pain. Or we think the patient thinks we are doing a good job if and when we do. It is a tricky business.

Pain, and often suffering, are wake-up calls. There are so many pain-management tools in this world. Or pain avoidance strategies. What if we ask ourselves, how is the pain HELPING this person? How can we as practitioners expand our consciousness to allow people to be in pain and not let it be reflective of the adequacy or inadequacy of our adjustment? If objective parameters are guiding our care, then the resolution or non-resolution of pain and suffering are secondary. I have heard practitioners say they get hyper-focused and upset at the process of trying to control people's pain. I have heard other practitioners say that in the first visit they tell people, "I do not fix pain. I do not want you to talk about your pain because that is not my focus." To be obsessed with controlling pain or adamant to not discuss it creates unnecessary polarity. Pain is important to listen to, for both the patient and the doctor. I have often referred people to other practitioners based upon what they told me about their pain and I continued to adjust them too. As I explained to the patient, more than one thing is going on here. You are subluxated AND you need the help of another professional.

As practitioners, we can benefit from gentle and wise

understanding of the level of consciousness the person is at, and allowing the process of chiropractic care to bring them up the ladder of consciousness. As vertebral subluxation clears, the brain changes. The patient now has the opportunity to evolve as life unfolds. In my personal experience, chiropractic care allowed me to travel up the rungs of the ladder of consciousness from numbness to suffering to wanting to live as much as possible through connection to my source of life. It is through this lens that I view ripple waves of "alivening" through my community. As Chiropractic evolves and matures, may we continue to honour the magnitude of the expression of life over a clear nervous system. May the alivening that happens in all of our offices ripple through the universe.

Ryan Carlson DC

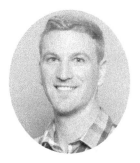

Dr Ryan Carlson graduated from chiropractic school at Northwestern Health Sciences University in 2016. He has since built one of the largest chiropractic health centres in the state of Arkansas, where he currently adjusts and changes the lives of over 400 patients a week. A success which he only has visions of expanding in the future.

Going to pharmacy school before Chiropractic School, Dr Carlson has seen all sides of healthcare. For that reason, he strives to spread the message of true health and healing through Chiropractic to those in his community, teaching with Dr Brad Glowaki on 4 different continents every year to keep the profession moving forward.

Breaking the limits for the future of Chiropractic

It was 6 May, 1954 at Oxford University's Iffley Road Track in Oxford, England. The 25-year-old Roger Bannister didn't know it at the time, but he was about to make history. For decades, middle-distance runners had scoffed at the idea that running a 4-minute mile was humanly possible. Those who thought otherwise were regarded as omnipotent and weren't taken seriously.

But Roger Bannister didn't believe in placing limitations on himself. He was on a mission to prove the ridiculers wrong, and he did so on that day when he ran the race in 3:59.4. Since then, over 1,400 individuals have broken the 4-minute mile barrier, the first of which occurred just 2 months later.

The same original type of small thinking has plagued many kingdoms, countries, professions, and individuals since the beginning of time. Limiting beliefs have been holding back mankind for centuries and even thousands of years, since the very first humans walked across the earth.

We all struggle with this from time to time and DD Palmer, the discoverer of Chiropractic, was likely no exception. But he was also innately intuitive, and consistently questioned the thoughts and ideas of those around him. Learning the art of magnetic healing from a great mentor of his, DD was raised to think differently from those in mainstream medicine at the time, and in so doing was able to change healthcare forever, with the discovery of the profession we all know and love, Chiropractic.

During my time in chiropractic school, I would often think of what went through DD's head in the months and years leading up to 1895, and exactly how he came to discover the subluxation and bringing about the correction of it through the adjustment.

No doubt he had many different ideas and tried numerous healing arts in his search for the cure of dis-ease.

Each time he would have a little idea, a tiny "thot flash," essentially something that he had to experiment with. The lesson to learn from all of this is that these small ideas are crucial to listen to, because without small ideas tested over time, a big idea can never come into fruition. DD's little idea about pushing on Harvey Lillard's back turned into the big idea we all know and cherish today, and it's all thanks to DD listening to his innate.

When we trust our innate intelligence to provide us with the answers we need, we are able to innovate. Yes, trusting our innate leads us to innovate! DD was in tune with his innate intelligence on that day in September, 1895 when he was 50 years old. How many 50-year-old individuals are still searching for truth and meaning today? Most at 50 are beginning to think of their retirement, as they mindlessly grind out another week.

It's true that chiropractors have always been different, clearly displayed by the Palmer family. Chiropractors who truly understand the philosophy of what we do have always questioned the mainstream; mainstream medicine, mainstream media, mainstream food, even mainstream fashion (BJ's cape was not the typical businessman's attire of the day!). I say we need to embrace this. The world needs individuals to think differently, and why shouldn't it be those who are more in touch with their innate intelligence than anyone; chiropractors and our well-adjusted individuals.

What we cannot lose sight of in this profession is our tribes; our patients. Through proper communication skills, education, and the untethering of limiting beliefs in our patients' minds, we can change the health culture of our communities, countries, and eventually our world. In order to do this, chiropractors must break through their own limitations within our philosophy. For the chiropractors reading this, do you truly go into your practice every day expecting miracles? When someone rolls into your office in a wheelchair, do you envision the same person walking out of your office one day? When someone tells you of the 27 medications he is taking daily, do you foresee the day that he takes none?

During my last year of chiropractic school, I decided I never wanted to put limitations on Chiropractic. After seeing what it had already done for me at that time, and after hearing of all the miracles other chiropractors and patients had seen and experienced, I tattooed BJ's famous words on my forearm: "Expect Miracles". You see, if you expect something, it's not negotiable, it's not a maybe; it's expected. I wanted to make sure that I was reminded of this with every single adjustment, as that quote is the last thing I see on my forearm before I adjust every one of my patients.

Chiropractors have expected great things and have worked through limitations brilliantly since the beginning. DD Palmer created a new healing art and expected many people to benefit from it; an account tells of 91 patients seated in his reception room waiting for his 1pm practice opening time. BJ Palmer expected to make Chiropractic a world-class profession; he owned the first car ever west of the Mississippi River and later bought a BJ Palmer Clinic ambulance to rush patients to his office. Clarence Gonstead expected to reach hundreds of thousands; he built an airport and motel for his practice in rural Wisconsin. Minora Paxson was a female who wanted to practice Chiropractic during a time when gender roles were less than favourable for her; she was the first female chiropractor and graduated from DD Palmer's School and Cure in 1900. She became a faculty member at 2 chiropractic colleges and co-authored the very first textbook on Chiropractic. Females have been highflyers in Chiropractic since the profession was founded.

Although there were only 12,000 practicing chiropractors in the first 30 years, there were 15,000 prosecutions for "practicing medicine without a licence". Many of their patients would picket outside the jails with signs that said, "We want our Doctor!" Chiropractors have been fighters since the profession was created, and have not let resistance stop them. Where many professions facing that amount of pressure would have caved numerous times, Chiropractic has survived, and now the time is right to go beyond survive, and begin to truly thrive!

Now, this isn't to say we haven't had our fair share of challenges. Many over the years have tried to limit us to neck pain and back pain; a portion of our profession still wants prescription rights; more and more chiropractors are focusing on modalities rather than the life-giving adjustment; and the American Medical Association has tried to end Chiropractic permanently, numerous times in the past. These challenges have brought confusion for chiropractic students and recent grads, and divisions have occurred time and time again.

My plea to those who influence our students and young graduates, is that we don't forget about our roots as a profession, that we don't forget about those who have risked it all and gone to jail so that we can still adjust and turn on nervous systems today, and that we don't forget the limitations that those before us have fought through. Even though it was only 125 years ago, the world was a very different place when DD delivered the first adjustment. Motor vehicles were all but non-existent, the calculator was 70 years from creation, and very little was truly known about the human body. Yet DD was so far ahead of his time in his thinking that he first voiced ideas that are only recently being proved by modern day research.

Therefore, let's not put limits on what Chiropractic can and cannot do for the body. Let's no longer try to "fit in" with medicine; that's a dying system, and we need to continue to promote a different, safer, more effective model to the public. Let's no longer hold onto neck pain and back pain, but let's intelligently promote our vitalistic roots by sharing what we know about the power of a properly-functioning nervous system. In the early 1900s, chiropractors used to advertise by including "No Questions Asked" on their promotional material, essentially meaning that what the patient had to share about symptoms was of less importance than what the spine and nervous system was showing. The early chiropractors were so confident that they could remove the subluxation, and that anything was possible when the body was at ease.

We truly have a simple message: if the body's nervous system is not working well, then the body cannot work well either, but if the body's nervous system is functioning properly, the body will trend that way too. This should be common sense within the healthcare fields, but where Chiropractic has made unparalleled strides is with the intimate relationship between this same nervous system and the spine. And a glorious relationship it is! Let's not forget to hold onto it, or some other profession will finally catch up and latch on.

It is predicted that even the most isolated individual will

influence over 10,000 people in his or her lifetime. Whether student, chiropractor, or chiropractic admirer, just imagine what we can accomplish if we all push to get the message of true health and healing out there. It won't be easy, because criticism is the price we pay for influence – the more influence you have, the more critics you'll have as well – but it's worth it to change a lost world.

Most people don't accidentally do a lot of good for the world. It takes intentionality. Choose to be intentional with every interaction you have, with every adjustment you give, and with everything you do for this profession. Don't put limits on Chiropractic, because it's Chiropractic that has kept limits off you.

Wisdom #14

Amy Spoelstra DC

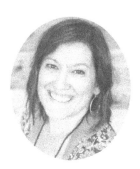 *Amy is the founder of the FOCUS program and Neuro-Deflective Retraining Method ™, FOCUS educational seminars for chiropractors, FOCUS Academy ™ and the Brain Blossom Program ™. Alongside being in practice, she has been helping children and adults with neurodevelopmental disorders since 2011.*

Amy is also co-founder of Navigate Your Healing, designed to help families who are affected by neurodevelopmental disorders. She and her husband David live in Coeur d'Alene with their beautiful daughter, Meela, and chocolate lab, Izzy with whom they love to travel.

Answer the call

"We chiropractors work with the subtle substance of the soul. We release the prisoned impulse, the tiny rivulet of force that emanates from the mind and flows over the nerves to the cells and stirs them into life." - BJ Palmer, DC, PhC, 1949

There was a boy, a girl, a mother, and a father. There was stress. There was growth. There was struggle.

This boy was "just being a boy," the mom was told. This boy would "grow out of it". This boy "is fine".

This boy "needs more discipline", the mom was told. The pain in his stomach is "normal". His frustration is "normal".

This boy is "lazy". He will "catch up in the future". The

mom is called "too sensitive". "Take these medications," the mother was told. It's "normal".

Slowly, it became painstakingly clear that none of it was actually "normal" or "fine" or "grown out of" or "caught up." That's when the mother and father said, what else is available?

Who can help? Why is he struggling? Why are we ALL struggling?

Who is there to answer this call with logic, understanding, compassion, science, and results? Who is there to make a case for healthy development and function, not solely from an old, established system of beliefs, but, instead, an understanding of what the science tells us now? Who is there and can listen and provide information, understanding, and support?

Broader questions emerge.

How many of these boys and girls and moms and dads live in every community around the globe? How many families need someone to answer this call?

Way too many.

This is the story of a typical family, my family, and the path of challenge and hardship that led me to the destination of Chiropractic.

What if someone had been able to speak to my family about how the response to stress in the body could lead to vast changes in the trajectory of brain development and alter the way a child develops and therefore alter his life? What if my family knew this in the moment it was first needed?

What if someone was capable of explaining to my parents that this response to stress (that alters efficient neurological function) can alter development and result in changes in the way a child learns, engages and connects with their world now and throughout life?

What if a chiropractor could bridge the gap between the challenges my brother was having and the impact of subluxation on the developing brain, directly and in an educated, unemotional way?

What if a chiropractor could make a case to a parent (who is currently experiencing fear, stress, and decision fatigue) that removing subluxation can impact the developing brain? Not by professing or implying that Chiropractic would cure or treat the neurodevelopmental disorder their child is experiencing. Nor by stating or believing that Chiropractic should be the only tool in the tool bag for this child. Instead, how about we create a foundation of healthy neurological function to till the soil for everything that comes next?

What would that have meant for my family? What would that mean to the family down the road from you, with the toddler struggling to develop expressive language or the teenager who is having trouble making social connections and struggles with depression? Perhaps that teenager is impacted by deflected development that began as a response to stress? Stress that altered the trajectory of growth and impaired the tools needed to connect with his or her world and make meaningful connections with peers.

We need to connect the dots for families and individuals who are struggling to live a healthy expression of life. I believe we have a responsibility to give them another option to consider, instead of just waiting for them to "grow out of it" or rely solely on one paradigm to cover symptoms, routinise behaviors, and expand weaknesses. We need to be able to ask and answer the big questions as they relate to individuals with behavioral, learning, socialisation, and developmental challenges. These questions fall into 2 categories:

1. How is this child (or adult) processing their world? What tools are they using to connect, engage, and learn from their environment? What does that tell us about the trajectory of development and the architecture of the developing brain?

2. Is there evidence of anything impacting the way the brain is receiving, processing, integrating, and sending information that may impact the way a child can move through development appropriately and efficiently?

We have a responsibility to understand more about development and how to work with families and individuals (also the medical and scientific world) to be a part of the solution. We do that by learning more, asking questions, taking ego out of the equation, and observing the wide array of developmental patterns that can lead to impaired function.

To do this, we must explore 3 main areas:

Our philosophy

In our profession, we understand that an individual is more than the sum of its parts. We are guided by the philosophy that we cannot simply have one symptom or presentation, without it being connected to the whole. Each symptom or "part" gives us a clue to the bigger picture of how a person's body is functioning, healing, adapting (or NOT adapting). We are clear that there may be many individuals suffering from the same symptom of back pain, for example, but the cause may be down to a variety of reasons. It is not our responsibility to cover, treat, cure, or relieve that symptom. It is our responsibility to understand it, as it is a window into the body.

We are then tasked with identifying underlying inefficiencies that may or may not be causing the symptom directly, but which are certainly contributing to the function of the whole person. The secondary sign of pain is not what we are chasing; it is merely a window into the body's current state. The condition we look for and correct, to improve underlying inefficient neurological function, is of course vertebral subluxation. We locate, analyse, and correct subluxation because we know its impact on the whole of the being's function. We are confident, mostly, in this understanding and application as it relates to a healthy individual or an individual with musculoskeletal symptoms.

However, when it comes to behavioral, learning, and socialisation challenges, even the most principled chiropractors tend to quickly shift from a "whole to part approach" to attempting to treat the behavior or deficit (symptom). As a profession, we tend to use the symptom or behavior as the sole marker of progress and effectiveness of correcting subluxation in this demographic. For instance, it is easy to jump to another modality and lose the clarity of the value of correcting subluxation, if a child's hyperactive behavior is still present after a period of time.

It is essential to use neurological function measurements, integrate observational tools, and conduct thorough clinical exams to witness that the behavior is a window into the brain of the individual. Maintaining our role as a chiropractor working in the "expression of life" model, as opposed to treating the symptoms of Neuro–Deflective Disorders, allows us to be a critical and foundational part of the team. This enables us to not become another therapy in the mechanistic paradigm that we do subscribe to. It is imperative to many of these kids and adults that we are a part of the team and perhaps not the only team member.

Simplify the Clinical Approach

In order to do the greatest good, it is important that we work from a "whole to part" perspective, both philosophically and clinically. In my clinical experience, I have found it helpful to utilise a clinical, hierarchical approach to ask and answer the big questions mentioned above, namely, "How is this child (or adult) processing their world?" and "Is there evidence of anything impacting the way the brain is receiving information?"

Utilising hierarchies of development allows us to have a clinical road map. This sets the foundation for the chiropractor to evaluate critically, perform an appropriate case history, perform accurate exams, make proper recommendations for care, create appropriate goals, and establish effective working relationships with other professionals, while staying grounded in the science, art, and philosophy of our own profession. It allows us to have ease in communication with providers that may be critical to the team for our patients such as neuro-optometrists, occupational therapists, educators, parents, speech therapists, and other medical providers. When we can boil down the complexity of neurodevelopment and understand and educate on the role that efficient neurological function plays on the developing brain, it becomes clear at times it must be "us and other providers", and not, "us or them."

Create a safe place to land

An often overlooked and quickly pushed aside consideration for effectively working with individuals with behavioral, learning, socialisation, and developmental challenges is the understanding of the neurology of the caretakers, decision-makers, or parents of the kids you are aiming to serve. You must first create a safe place for caregivers/parents with your office procedures, and your verbal and non-verbal communication.

While easily overlooked, striving to complete this piece of the puzzle may be one of the most important and impactful parts of the journey in building a practice and profession, for improving the expression of life for those with neurodevelopmental disorders. These parents/caretakers are often in a state of chronic stress, over-stimulation, and decision fatigue. As a business, your establishment must continually work to understand how to engage and communicate with an individual in chronic stress, while simultaneously meeting the need of the patient who is likely in a different neurological state to the caretaker. While this can seem very intimidating, the reality is that you can use the same hierarchical understanding to determine the needs of the parents/caregivers as you do for the patient, and easily learn to adapt the environment and demand, to meet them both appropriately.

If you don't create a safe place to land for your patients and their families, you may never have the opportunity to open the door to help. You must demonstrate through your actions, procedures, and communication that you think differently about their child and family. You will likely find you are the only provider or business that has ever taken steps to see and interact with their child and not just their child's deficit.

With that said, what if we were able to do this in all of our communities around the globe? Imagine if we were able to create a safe place to land and allow philosophical and clinical excellence to be the foundation for improving the expression of life for kids and adults with deflected development and processing patterns. We have the ability to impact the way children learn, engage, and connect with their world. We not only have an opportunity, but a responsibility to be the ones to answer the call to families like my own family.

The gift we have been given to be a part of the solution, to release the mental impulse, to impact the trajectory of one life, is one I will never take lightly and I am honoured to be surrounded by others who are also drawn to the call.

Do you remember the boy who was "just being a boy", and would "grow out of it?"

I know I was put on this earth to do this work; the struggle has led to clarity and growth. Will you join me and answer the call?

Steve Williams DC DC, DICS, FICS, FRCC (paeds), FBCA

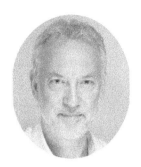

Steve Williams DC has practiced for 33 years with a special interest in paediatrics. He is a sought-after speaker, lecturer and teacher as well as author of the widely acclaimed book Pregnancy and Paediatrics: A Chiropractic Approach. Steve is currently Vice President of the BCA and has served on the regulatory board for the General Chiropractic Council in London. He has been President of SOTO Europe and SOTO International and was a founding board member of the Royal College of Chiropractic Paediatric Faculty.

As well as teaching his popular paediatrics course around the world, Steve has developed and taught paediatrics courses at AECC, Madrid and Barcelona Chiropractic College.

Chiropractic- Maximising A Child's Potential

My story about Chiropractic is somewhat unusual, in that during my first years of Chiropractic I was terrified of babies, and now I'm known as a paediatric chiropractor. In a way it chose me, rather than me choosing it, which is something that happens in life, perhaps showing a degree of pre-destination.

That journey began with the birth of my son Tom, when I was in my first year of practice. This gorgeous baby was a refluxing, vomiting, crying nightmare, following a difficult entry into the world. His birth was induced and he became stuck in the birth canal for many hours, eventually coming out with a moulded ring around his head and a startled look in his eyes.

He cried non-stop, was a slow developer, difficult to put down at any stage as a baby and had to wear thick "bottle-top" glasses by 18 months of age. I could see where the long-term outcomes were going; he would be a slow-developing, poorly-attaining, hyperactive, clumsy child and I thought Chiropractic must be able to do something to alter this course. So, I went everywhere I could think of, both in the UK and the US, learning from the best. Gradually and progressively, many of his problems improved. By 6 or 7 he was out of glasses and improving at school. By 15 years he was on the verge of international schoolboy rugby, which just seemed incredible for a boy who had been a severely dyspraxic child. He became head boy of his senior school, got a good degree and went on to qualify as a chartered accountant. He is now a senior accountant at a FTSE 100 company. My belief is that without chiropractic care he would never have attained anywhere near this in life, so my chiropractic future was chosen for me. I had to help other children similarly affected to have the same opportunity to fulfil their potential.

We see so many infants with poor tone, structural asymmetry, plagiocephaly, slow development, gastrointestinal problems, autonomic dysfunction (often parasympathetic inhibition) and a raft of other problems. If these are not addressed in early infancy, long term problems often follow such as an asymmetry of brain development associated with neurodevelopmental disorders. Infants with poor tone and structural asymmetry, for example positional head preference from upper cervical subluxation,[1] will often be slow developing or asymmetric in the development of the cerebellar-thalamo-cortical loops, causing one cerebral hemisphere to develop poorly, compared to the other.

Right hemisphere deficiency is associated with ADHD,

---

1 Biedermann H JMPT 2005:28;e1-e15

autistic spectrum disorders and obsessive-compulsive disorders, among other problems. Left hemisphere deficiency is associated with dyslexia and other learning disorders[2]. Early signs that infants may be heading for significant cortical asymmetry include being slow for dates with gross motor skills such as rolling, sitting up, crawling and walking, retaining their neonatal or primitive reflexes significantly longer than they should and major feeding problems.

Infants with gastrointestinal problems, for example reflux, colic or constipation will often be put on medications such as proton pump inhibitors or hydrogen receptor antagonists. These drugs are associated with gastrointestinal and respiratory infections, increased (30%) fracture risk and small intestine bacterial overgrowth (SIBO)[3][4,5]. The sequelae to this can be a lifetime of gut issues with a less diverse microbiome and a leaky gut, where the widespread interstitial spaces that young infants have to absorb the maternal immunoglobulins don't close down to the tight junctions between the cells that they should. This may well be a cause of later auto-immune dysfunction and food sensitivities, as over-large molecules of various foods are absorbed, often leading to antibody-antigen reactions.

Autonomic imbalance, particularly sympathetic dominance, is associated with a very twitchy, easily disturbed baby who may well show an exaggerated Moro or startle reflex. This may be a result of the maternal stress response being heightened and sensitising the foetus's, and later the infant's, system to adrenaline and cortisol. Even such seemingly unrelated issues

2 Melillo R Disconnected Kids Penguin Putnam 2010
3 Malchodi et al Pediatrics 2019 Jul;144(1):
4 Cohen et al Br J Clin Pharmacol. 2015 Aug;80(2):200–8
5 Rosen et al J Pediatr Gastroenterol Nutr 2018 Mar;66(3):516–554

like adverse maternal childhood experiences have been linked to infant gastrointestinal dysfunction and poor bonding.

Direct mechanical vagal nerve dysfunction also probably plays a major part. The vagus nerve is vulnerable to interference by subluxations affecting the skull base, C0-C1, the sternoclavicular joint and the thoracolumbar junction and lower ribs, stressing the diaphragm.

Cranial nerve X (vagus) exits the jugular foramen along with cranial nerves IX (glossopharyngeal), XI (spinal accessory) and the jugular vein between the occiput and the temporal bones. The occiput is in 4 parts and the temporal in 3 parts at this stage and the jugular foramen is vulnerable to both compression and torsion in the birth process which often occur, creating vagal, glossopharyngeal and spinal accessory dysfunction.

Upper cervical subluxation (C0-C1), creating occipital condyle stress, can also noxiously affect the same cranial nerves. The vagus then passes under the medial clavicle where it can be vulnerable to inferior medial clavicle subluxations and then through the diaphragm where either mid cervical subluxations affecting the phrenic nerve or thoraco-lumbar and 12th rib subluxations can create diaphragm tension and subsequent vagal inhibition.

If the vagus nerve is inhibited, the sympathetic (fight or flight) nervous system becomes over expressed. This leads to the infant's sensory systems being constantly on alert, where everyday sounds, sights and movements can stimulate a Moro response. Each time this response occurs, the infant produces adrenaline and cortisol, shutting down digestion, sending blood to the skeletal muscles, increasing blood glucose and heightening the infant's senses. When this happens the food in the infant's gut stops being digested and is liable to start degrading, encouraging a less desirable microbiome and creating gut inflammation, poor immune function and increasing the infant's gastrointestinal issues. If this hyper-sympathetic responsiveness continues, the gut does not mature appropriately with a rich and diverse microbiome. A lifetime of gastrointestinal and inflammatory problems may well follow.

We know the development of the gut microbiota occurs primarily in infancy and is hugely involved in our long-term health outcomes, and I am convinced proper balance of the autonomic nervous system is essential to its development and not just the health of the gut but also our children's long-term health[6].

For me, the beauty of chiropractic paediatrics is that if we see the infant when young (within the first 3 months of its life preferably) we have a window of opportunity to correct the imbalance in their system relatively easily, before it becomes the norm for that child to have aberrant afferent firing patterns affecting brain development, showing as delayed milestones or inappropriate movement patterns.

For me, inspired by the incredible results in my own children, I will only be content when all infants are able to access expert chiropractic paediatric care in their first weeks or months of life. I believe that would hugely decrease the disease burden in society and allow more children to reach their potential and express the best parts of the best of their genetic makeup. It has become my passion to teach chiropractors how to treat babies and children, and to change their lives.

That experience with my son also taught me that while

---

6 Dinan and Cryan J Physiol. 2017 Jan 15;595(2):489-503

I expected to proceed in a particular direction life, fate or whatever you want to call it may have other ideas, and rather than fighting it, just go with it and in my experience, you will love the job.

Wisdom #15

Adrian Wenban BSC, BAppSc, MMedSc, PGrDip(Med Ed)DC

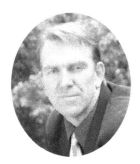 *Adrian Wenban is presently the Principal of the Barcelona College of Chiropractic. He holds a B.Sc. (Anatomy), a B.App.Sc. (Chiropractic), a M.Med.Sc. (Clinical Epidemiology) and a P. Gr.Cert. (Medical Education). In practice for more than 20 years, he has worked in 5 different countries and was the president of the Fundación Privada Quiropráctic from 2007 to 2009.*

Adrian's areas of interest include philosophy of science, curriculum development and reviewing peer-reviewed health care literature. He is a member of the Spanish Chiropractic Association (AEQ), the Australasian Epidemiology Association (AEA), the Chiropractic Association of Australia (CAA) and the Association for the Study of Medical Education (ASME).

Beyond the body as a machine, towards the body as intelligent

There is no avoiding the use of metaphors. Metaphors and models (which are also metaphors) lie at the heart of our everyday communication and our practice as chiropractors. The purpose of a metaphor is to take something we know and use it to explain something we don't. The word has its roots in the Greek metapherein, meaning to transfer or carry. By linking two disparate things, a metaphor carries some quality from one to the other. It takes the concreteness of something we can imagine and carries it to something we can't. However, there are some metaphors that are better avoided and others which, although useful at one point in time or in one context, may not always be of the greatest utility in communicating one's intended message.

Take for example, the *body as machine* metaphor. Out of humble beginnings in Greek philosophy, machine metaphors rose to a position of prominence and, in the 19th and 20th centuries, assumed great dominance in western science and healthcare (Vaccari, 2003). It could be argued that along the way, Descartes' Traité de l'homme (1662) was the most sophisticated articulation of the early modern machine-body and that it was the first extended attempt to rewrite life in strictly machine-like terms (Vaccari, 2003).

DD Palmer, the Founder of Chiropractic, positioned himself very clearly in relation to the utility of the machine metaphor when he said, "*To attempt to demonstrate the vital acts of the human body by the working of machinery is futile.*" Palmer went on to contend that, "*There is no similarity between living bodies which possess functions, and machines by which goods are manufactured.*"

Despite DD's appreciation of the limitations of the machine metaphor as far back as 1910, much of modern biology and healthcare, and indeed modern chiropractic education and research, is predicated on a mechanistic understanding of the human body. One where we view ourselves as carbon-based multicellular machines. By way of logical extension of that machine metaphor, we are drawn into seeing a doctor as a mechanic, whose job it is to find the broken, malfunctioning or worn-out parts and to remove, replace, fix, repair or supplant them when the body's limitations of matter are exceeded. For at least a century now, this has been the primary metaphor for healthcare providers and patients, to think and talk about disease and its absence. The effect on clinical problem solving and framing the healthcare encounter is all pervasive, so the care provider sees the patient as seeking his expertise and skill in repairing that which is broken, has failed, or is in need of repair/replacement. Inherent in this *body as machine* metaphor and resultant mechanical clinical encounter, an extension of Newton's Clockwork Universe, is that the body is fallible, flawed and without the resources to self-heal.

On many levels, the body as machine metaphor has served mankind. As Randolph Nesse, Professor of Life Sciences at Arizona State University's Centre for Evolution and Medicine points out: "The metaphor of body as a machine provided a ladder that allowed biology to bring phenomena up from a dark pit of mysterious forces into the light, where organic mechanisms can be analysed."

And so, as a result of the success of the machine metaphor, and despite its limitations, we now have a vast and detailed understanding of much of the function and mechanisms that underpin normal and aberrant human physiological and biochemical processes (Vaccari, 2003).

However, more recent advances are revealing that this central metaphor of both biology and medicine is limited and indeed, fundamentally flawed. Some of today's most important discoveries in areas of study such as epidemiology, epigenetics and neuroplasticity, have profoundly changed our understanding of phenomena like contextual healing, placebo and nocebo effects. Moreover, these discoveries undermine the utility of the machine metaphor and generate opportunity for advancing more useful clinical metaphors.

Two such metaphors which have a history of use in chiropractic are the metaphor of *body as terrain* and *body as intelligent.* Both have the potential to frame and underpin education, research and clinical practice models that would have chiropractic educationalists, researchers and practitioners asking different questions, communicating different understandings and providing care in different ways that might better align with the fundamental philosophical principles that ground chiropractic in offering something uniquely important in the care of patients (Coulter et al., 2019).

In *Metaphors We Live By, Lakoff,* a linguist and Johnson, a philosopher, suggest that metaphors not only make our thoughts more vivid and interesting but that they actually structure our perceptions and understanding. Metaphor is for most people a device of the poetic imagination and the rhetorical flourish. Moreover, metaphor is typically viewed as characteristic of language alone, a matter of words rather than thought or action. On the contrary, Lakoff and Johnson found that metaphor is pervasive in everyday life, not just in language but in thought and action. Our ordinary conceptual system, in terms of which we both think and act, is *"fundamentally metaphorical in nature"* *(Younis, 2016).*

In keeping with these findings, it can be argued that the clinical metaphors we adopt have real world implications. If we proceed in the clinical realm applying the metaphor of *body as intelligent,* as opposed to *body as machine,* we might choose to look at individual patients, presenting with some symptom profiles, very differently. Take for example the case of a pregnant women presenting with morning sickness.

Nausea and emesis in early pregnancy are common phenomena affecting as many as 70% of pregnant women but little is known about the aetiology and role of this common and often incapacitating bodily response. Within the medical community it is common for morning sickness to be thought of as a symptom of pregnancy, almost as if pregnancy were a disease. The logic, in dealing with this symptom from the *body as machine* metaphorical perspective seems to have been: morning sickness makes women uncomfortable, so let's alleviate the symptom, usually pharmacologically, and thereby relieve them of their discomfort. Many chiropractors also conceptualise their role such that they strive to help patients by relieving symptoms, like morning sickness, through chiropractic adjustments.

However, if we instead consider morning sickness from the *body as intelligent* perspective, we will instead seek to understand the origin of this bodily response and determine whether it serves an evolved and necessary function. Furthermore, doing so would surely be in keeping with our respect for the body's inherent self-regulating capacity. So, before attempting to mask this symptom, lets instead ask the question: "In generating morning sickness, is the body, on some level, doing exactly what is best for the foetus and/or mother to be?" A recent literature review (Flaxman, 2000), published in a peer-reviewed journal called Obstetrics & Gynecology finds considerable support for a theory, initially developed by an evolutionary biologist called Margie Profet, which speaks highly of the body's inborn intelligence.

Profet developed her theory based on some of the following research findings:

- A number of studies have now shown that women with morning sickness are less likely to suffer miscarriages or have premature or low birth weight babies.
- Women who vomit suffer fewer miscarriages than those who experience nausea alone.
- Women with no morning sickness symptoms have higher rates of miscarriage and underweight babies.
- Actively metabolising tissues are more vulnerable to toxins than dormant ones, cells that divide rapidly are more readily interfered with than quiescent ones, and cells that differentiate into specialised types are more susceptible than those that just reproduce more of the same.
- Morning sickness peaks when the embryonic organogenesis is most susceptible to chemical disruption (weeks 6-18).
- There is a close correlation between the time when the foetal liver is least able to detoxify many chemical compounds and when a pregnant women experiences morning sickness.
- There is a correlation between toxin concentrations and the tastes and odours that cause pregnant women to be nauseous.

Based on the above findings, and in keeping with the *body as intelligent* perspective, Profet asked, "Could it be that morning sickness is actually an example of the body's inborn wisdom expressing health exactly as it is designed to?"

Profet hypothesised that nausea and food aversions during the first trimester of pregnancy serve as important protective mechanisms for the developing foetus (Profet, 1996). She argued that morning sickness has evolved to impose dietary restrictions on the mother and thereby minimise foetal exposure to toxins while the developing liver is most unable to detoxify certain chemicals found in common foods. If Profet's hypothesis proved to be right it certainly would not make much sense to pharmaceutically interfere with the symptom of morning sickness.

Although the theory has undergone a number of revisions as more data has come to hand, it certainly now seems that morning sickness, which might be better thought of as "morning wellness", is important for optimal foetal development and wellbeing. A recent review by Flaxman and Sherman (2000), from the Department of Neurobiology and Behaviour at Cornell University, concluded that, "Available data are most consistent with the hypothesis that morning sickness serves an adaptive prophylactic function".

Without a doubt, the body's inborn wisdom knows best and as a result we should act in accordance with the conservative ethic aspired to by our forefathers that suggested we should "first do no harm". In the case of so-called morning sickness, what appeared, from a limited reductionistic perspective, to be an uncomfortable bodily malfunction, is instead proving in a broader sense, to be an essential foetal protective mechanism. We will do well to respect the inherent wisdom of living organisms. Two authors (Lumley, 1998; Huxley, 2000), in reviewing Profet's work, concluded, "...pregnant women should be extremely wary of ALL DRUGS, both therapeutic and recreational... Certainly, it would be wise to avoid taking any medication."

Other than avoiding drugs, what should a pregnant mother

do about her nausea? In short, respect it. This intelligent response to certain foods is an adaptive process, born from within, that increases the likely-hood of health for the next generation, both in utero and beyond.

Furthermore, because some symptoms such as morning sickness have an important health optimising function, we as chiropractors might do well to explore, clinically and scientifically, the extent of our role in helping the body to accurately interpret its environment, thereby generating the optimum adaptive response. We might best serve the evolved adaptive abilities of a patient by applying the *body as intelligent* as opposed to the less respectful, more dehumanizing, *body as machine* metaphor. Making the conscious decision not to attempt to minimise a woman's morning sickness seems counter intuitive at first. However, according to Profet's theory we will do well to avoid arrogantly assuming that morning sickness should be fixed, as if the body was malfunctioning. We might also help to improve the wellbeing of our species by further exploring the degree to which symptoms in general are an intelligent and appropriate response to internal and external environmental stimuli.

Lewis Thomas (Thomas, 1979), the former dean of both Yale and New York School of Medicine and president of Memorial Sloan-Kettering Institute, said, "*A kind of super intelligence exists in each of us, infinitely smarter and possessed of technical know-how, far beyond our present understanding.*"

Patrick Sim BSc, MChiro, DC

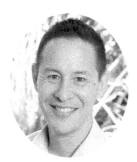

The inaugural CEO and President of the Australian Chiropractic College, Patrick graduated as a chiropractor in 1997 from Macquarie University in NSW. With over 20 years of practice experience, he has also amassed an additional 26 years of leadership in the profession.

Patrick has served with the Chiropractor's Association of Australia and registration boards. This experience has provided him with a unique view of the chiropractic profession that includes practitioner, professional and regulatory perspectives.

The Fourth Leg

I am not sure I agree with the whole thing of Chiropractic being a philosophy, science, and art, and I wonder if you might agree with me.

For this reason, I don't subscribe to the well-used "3 legs of a stool" metaphor to describe Chiropractic. The idea of a 3-legged stool has always struck me as an odd and unstable design. Most stools I've seen have either a single leg with a strong base, or 4 legs for stability. I wonder if the inherent instability of a 3-legged stool is mimicked in the plight of our profession over its existence, so I would like to argue for both the above models of the chiropractic stool.

I realise this might be a somewhat sacrilegious stance, as this triad is well embedded in chiropractic's identity, but one thing I have noticed in our profession is a propensity to subscribe to these axioms without question. While we don't need to obstreperously defy them, I believe a conscious process of consideration is required, especially when it comes to the bumper-sticker slogans in Chiropractic.

The idea of Chiropractic being philosophy, science and art is one such slogan often used, but I think poorly understood. To trot out the old war horse, Stephenson said in his 1927 text, *"Chiropractic is a philosophy, science and art of things natural; a system of adjusting the segments of the spinal column by hand only, for the correction of the cause of dis-ease (p. xiii),"* and sadly, this is where many stop reading.

If you were to read the remaining 15 lines of that passage and turn the page, you'd see that Stephenson goes on to say of the science, art, and philosophy of Chiropractic, that they are, *"what it is, how it is done, and why... science tells us what it is; art tells us how it is done, and philosophy, the "why" of the other two. According to that, then philosophy must tell us about both science and art..."*

When I read this, I take it to mean that when all is said and done, it is the philosophy which defines all that there is in Chiropractic. Without the philosophy, the science loses relevance, and the art loses its direction (excuse the pun), and I have to agree. The most important thing we have in Chiropractic is the philosophy. Before the science. Before the art. Too often the emphasis is placed on research and practical application, and only lip service paid to the raison d'être. This is not to say that research and the exquisite application of force are not worthy endeavours, but the pursuit of each to the detriment of the philosophy is a fool's game.

This is the argument for the single-legged stool with a strong base model. I am certainly not the first person to make this statement. In fact, I'd be surprised if I was the only one in this book saying this, but I may be able to provide a unique perspective on just how much I believe it, and what I am willing to do to defend it.

Here in Australia, we have been facing an extinction event. In fact, Australia has the worst mammalian extinction rate in the world, having lost 10% of its native mammals since the arrival of Europeans. In total there are 1,800 species of native Australian fauna and flora listed as critically endangered. But it is not only the fauna and flora of Australia that is in danger of extinction, it is also Chiropractic that faces this end. This is not because there is a lack of chiropractors in Australia either. The 4 university-based programmes churn out around 400 graduates per year. The problem is that very few of those graduates truly understand what Chiropractic is, and when I say Chiropractic, I mean the philosophy.

These graduates are good academics who understand science and they know methods of "treatment" (a dirty word as far as I am concerned) but have no professional identity, no sense of self or purpose. This leads to poor practitioners who fail in practice and spend their careers trying to justify their existence as a manual therapist. The bell curve of the profession in Australia indicates a greater alignment with physiotherapy and exercise science more than it does with true chiropractic practice.

This is then amplified in our representative bodies when these graduates take on positions of power or go back to teaching, worsening the problem by feeding back into the production of poorer graduates. Effectively, this is a process of eugenics; the breeding out of Chiropractic in Australia.

It was because of this that myself and 3 colleagues set about establishing a philosophically congruent, vitalistic chiropractic college that is scientifically rigorous, academically strong, with a keen business development stream in Australia, the Australian Chiropractic College. Strangely, the drive was actually not to create a college, that was just a means to an end. Our drive was to protect principles, tenets and philosophies that make Chiropractic distinct, effective, and sustainable, so future Australians will have access to it. We had to protect the philosophy. The government wasn't doing it. The association certainly wasn't doing it. No one was defending the *principle* in any meaningful or sustainable way. Without protection, Chiropractic was on the road to homogenisation as a manual therapy, and oblivion.

So, this is exactly what we did. We positioned people into representative bodies; we thoroughly examined legislation, constitutions, and laws; we hired experts and consultants; we formed strong international bonds that lead to the formation of our curriculum (thanks NZCC!) and, when we were ready, we launched our idea to the profession. Since that launch in 2016, we have raised $2million AUD, gained government approval, hired a stunning professional and academic team, secured a premises, and, on 28 January 2020, started teaching to ACC's first ever students. All of this can be summarised in one word, we played *politics*.

This brings me to the next model of the stool I want to present, the stability of the fourth leg. What is not recognised in the classic triad is the role of politics in chiropractic, the role of group action towards a common goal that defines laws within a society.

And don't tell me we would be better off without politics in Chiropractic! How you market and promote your practice is politics, the legislation you operate in was created through politics, your decision not to engage in politics is in fact your own politics in action. The Australian Chiropractic College would not have gotten off the ground if it were not for politics. It may still fail because of politics, and the Scotland College of Chiropractic will live or die due to politics. Our profession needs to recognise that there is a fourth leg to the stool, the leg of politics and that we must all engage with it. Clear politics provides stability and certainty. The greats of our profession, such as BJ and Reggie, all knew this and leveraged on that understanding to move the profession forward.

Another of our profession's great politicians, Dr Gerry Clum, once said, *"Your right at the adjusting table is earned by other people's blood sweat and tears at the negotiation table"*. He was dead right. Our ability to practice Chiropractic should never be taken for granted. It has been a long, hard road with many fights along the way. Too few of us are thankful enough to those who paved the way.

But there is a fickle flip-side to this too. The people you allow to represent you at the negotiation table will define you.

The reason that chiropractic in Australia is in its current state, is because too few people took the jump out of practice to serve the profession when it was needed. And right now, all around the world, the profession needs you.

Life in practice is comfortable and rewarding but when you look at it critically, it is self-serving. Yes, you can argue that you are serving the people of your community, but it is a very transactional level of service. I ask you to step out of that life and play a bigger game, really make a difference in the world by adding your passion for Chiropractic to a cause larger than yourself. Sometimes this level of service is in the form of your time; you can sit on late night meetings, write the boring submissions, read the legislation. But often what is really needed is the greatest political force you have, your money.

So often we play small in our lives. Dave Russell was one who did not. He dreamed of chiropractic education revitalising the profession. He recognised the problems many chiropractic programmes pose to Chiropractic and he wanted to address that head-on, through a new programme in Scotland. Now that he is gone, we all need to step up to take on part of the role he played and be bigger with our lives.

When we recognise that the fundamental essence of Chiropractic is its philosophy, and when we acknowledge that concerted action with honed political will informed by this philosophy is critical to our survival, all of chiropractic will see the benefits. For it is political force drawing on strong philosophy that ultimately changes the world. But what we must truly remember is that all of this discourse is for nothing, if we forget the purpose of a stool; for sitting. May the people we serve, our families and communities, know that whenever they need it, they may rest easy on the stool of chiropractic.

Wisdom #16

Russ Rosen DC

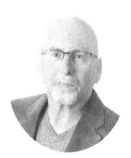

A dynamic and passionate chiropractor, author, international coach, educator and speaker, Russ ran one of the most successful wellness practices in Maui, Hawaii for 14 years. He is best known for his "Patient Care" vs "Patient Scare" Wellness Communication systems.

Russ has served as Lead Author and Director of Dr. Patrick Gentempo's Creating Wellness Management System and is also the proud recipient of CLA/CWA's 2007 "Lifetime Achievement" award. Since 2000 Russ has helped hundreds of doctors thrive in a True Optimal-Health model and is CEO of The Optimal Health Coaching System.

Principles

Here are some principles I hold near and dear when coaching chiropractors:

First principle

It is "Innate Intelligence" not "Innate Stupidity". Look through the lens of, "Why would innate intelligence do that? Why would innate wisdom cause that swelling, inflammation, pain or even cancer?" When we realise that innate is always doing its best to do the lesser of two evils or to choose life, it gives us a very different perspective.

I live by the principle, "When you clarify the problem, the solution becomes self-evident." When we look through the lens of innate intelligence not innate stupidity, it helps us to better help our patients.

Second principle

Disease care or sick care vs. healthcare. They have two different intents and purposes. The intent of disease/sick care is the detection and treatment of symptoms, disease and infirmity. The best you can hope for it to feel better. It is fixing the problem after it occurs. It is brilliant in emergency care and "fighting" some diseases and illnesses. But it has nothing to do with healthcare, prevention or wellness. You can be an MD, DC or any type of practitioner and practice in this model. Unfortunately, most DC's practice in this model, treating symptoms.

Disease is seen as the presence of something evil. In the 1700's, English sailors would go off on their ships and come back with their teeth falling out and bleeding gums. Because they believed these sailors had evil spirits, they burned them at the stake. And did that fix the problem? Yes, they no longer bled, after they were burned at the stake!

Later it was discovered that if they just gave the sailors a lime a day, they stopped having these terrible bleeding problems. Ergo the name, Limeys. Of course, the problem was not evil spirits. It was the absence of vitamin C.

In these modern times the drugs, machines and technologies have certainly advanced from burning you at the stake, bloodletting and giving you arsenic, but they are still going to war with the evil perpetrator causing your symptoms.

In the health and wellness model disease is not the presence of something evil, it is the absence of something essential. Give the body clean air, water, good food, exercise, mental health and a properly functioning nervous system and in the vast majority of cases people will thrive and be healthy. If you give the person the essential thing they are missing, they have the best chance of getting healthy and staying healthy. In Chiropractic we give them proper nerve supply and many of us help with lifestyle advice.

Again, neither is better than the other. They just have different intents and purposes. In my healthcare talk I would say, "If I am skydiving and my parachute does not open, and I happen to live, don't bring me to a healthcare provider like me. Bring me to the emergency room so they can stop the bleeding and put my bones back together."

But, if you want to get healthy and stay healthy, you really need to see one of the many wonderful healthcare providers, like me!

Third principle

This is one of the most important and powerful concepts I can get across to my coaching clients, which can set them free to get the best results, be the best doctor they can be, decrease their stress and thrive like never before. Yes, this is a biggie: Certainty is key. You must absolutely be certain that you CANNOT help everyone!

What?! He is a heretic!! Hang in there with me. Here is the challenge. We all hear that you MUST have certainty. We hear the gurus from the pulpit at our wonderful Rah Rah seminars say, "If I give them an adjustment, they are getting better!" They may also add, "Their symptoms may not go away, but if I adjust them, they are getting healthier, period!"

Really? Is that really true?

Here is the problem with that. We buy into the story that Chiropractic helps everyone. But when I ask doctors, and I have literally asked thousands of doctors at seminars and my one-on-one coaching clients if they have ever had a patient that they realised was just not improving under their care? Not symptomatically, not their X-rays, or scans, or myotomes, or whatever objective tests they use? And nearly 100% of them sheepishly look around the room before raising their hands, or if we are on a one-to-one coaching call, they almost whisper that they have had patients who have not done well under their care.

How about you? Have you had some patients who did not do well under your care? Of course you have! Unless of course you can walk on water!

So now, either chiropractic is a lie, or you suck! Which one of those certainties leads to growing a tremendous practice? Neither.

Is it possible that maybe your technique is not the right technique for this patient, and they would be better off seeing someone else? Or that without a particular nutrient, or changing their diet, or their job, they simply cannot get better? That your adjustments just will not hold or work for them? What if they are just not ready to heal? What if their karma is that they haven't hit rock bottom yet and they need to?

What I am saying is, that although I get the rhetoric, I used to say the same thing too. The reality is that some people are not going to do well under your care.

Once you acknowledge that with yourself and with your

patients, you can free yourself to swing for the fences, without the "what if I am not able to help this one?" That can be devastating to so many of us.

In our consultation we let the patient know: "My main goal is to see if you are in the right place to get the care that you need. And my promise is, I am going to help you. I am either going to recognise that I am the right doctor for you, or, if I feel I am not, I will do my best to refer you to someone who can help you. But I will not waste your time or money. Does that sound fair to you?"

In our report of findings, we let them know that we will monitor them very closely with our re-evaluations and re-reports. I personally let them know that I have a 3-visit rule. If I see you come back 3 times in a row with the same subluxation pattern, and it does not look like it is changing, either you need to do something differently (eat better, exercise, deal with stress) or I need to do something differently (possibly change techniques). We need to do something differently. Or I need to refer you out.

Please be clear, I am not saying, if they don't feel better within 3 visits. I am saying if they don't come back showing some objective improvement. Again, that is just how I practice. I am not trying to lay that on you. Each technique and person is different. I personally know that the body has amazing regenerative properties when we are doing the right things for our patients and we will see objective changes in the right direction as well as eventually subjective/symptomatic changes.

Once you get that agreement you can just go for it. And I promise you better results and more honest certainty and less stress!

Fourth principle

You cannot TELL anyone anything. No one wants to be educated. And the last thing they care about is Chiropractic.

The neuroscience of communications tells us that all information is filtered through the reptilian brain. And 95-99% of it does not make it up to the neocortex for thinking, reasoning and problem solving.

If we want our information, or our chiropractic story, to make it past the reptilian brain's filter so it gets to the neocortex for thinking and reasoning, (and assuming our story makes sense, and thank God, Chiropractic makes sense) and then get dropped into the limbic system as a new belief system, we must stop trying to TELL our patients anything. We need to start asking.

The neuroscience of communications tells us that the reptilian brain is there for survival. Food, fighting and fornication (not great things to do with our patients!)

If we want our information to get past the reptilian brain's filter we must make our story new, novel and exciting. And we must make it about them. We must make our story about them vs. trying to tell them OUR story.

We do this through Socratic questions. A Socratic question is a question that makes people think and come up with their own answers and own conclusions. Such as why do you think these headaches keep coming back and have not resolved. Versus, let me tell you why your headaches keep coming back and have not been resolved.

Now of course, we are going to teach them along the way, so they know how to answer those questions. But the art and skill of communications is not telling or educating. The skill to getting our patients to truly understand the value of our care and shift their consciousness or paradigm, is by learning how to ask the right questions. Which of course our entire communications course is built upon.

Fifth Principle

As Oscar Wilde said: *"Be yourself: everyone else is already taken."*

Your patients are looking for authenticity. When studying and learning from coaches like myself and other mentors, do everything you can to customise the materials and make them work for you.

I tell my clients they will never be as good at being me as I am. And I will never be as good at being them as they are. Be yourself. Make it your own. Be authentic. Always be ethical and tell the truth. Dogs and bees can smell fear and people can smell when you are not being authentic.

The truth is, in the end, if your patients do not buy YOU, they will not buy Chiropractic, or your recommendations.... I hope that helps.

Simon Senzon MA, DC, PhD (Candidate)

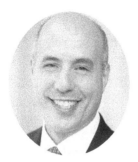

Simon is a 1999 Sherman Graduate. He is a PhD candidate at Southern Cross University's School of Health and Human Sciences, in Australia. His dissertation examines the flaws and strengths of the chiropractic literature as an Intellectual Field. He is the founder of The Institute Chiropractic, an online learning resource for the profession. He lives and practices in Asheville, North Carolina.

His recent books are DD Palmer: A Biography, and The Chiropractic Green Books: A Definitive Guide, and recent papers include The Morikubo Trial: A Content Analysis and the 10-part series on The Chiropractic Vertebral Subluxation.

Chiropractic's Grand Tradition

Throughout chiropractic history, there were a few chiropractors who exemplified the best in the profession. I don't mean the charismatic technique leaders, the heads of schools, or the well-known speakers on the circuit. Although, it's possible for these rare individuals to embody any or all those positions. I refer to the chiropractors who taught, practiced, researched, published, and built meaningful chiropractic relationships and collaborations; chiropractors like Dr David Russell.

Dr Russell was unique in Chiropractic because he was a scholar, a practitioner, a researcher and a teacher. He published over 25 papers, many of which were co-authored. Dave lived and breathed Chiropractic. He practiced, taught at a college for several years, and spoke at many conferences. I place him on the pedestal of exemplary chiropractors not only because of all these activities but because of who he was behind the scenes. He was a friend to many, a jovial colleague, and a tireless reviewer and editor of countless papers. It was this last attribute where I appreciated Dave immensely.

In the last 20 years I have published 16 books and dozens of articles on the science, art, history, and philosophy of Chiropractic. One of the most significant challenges for me as a chiropractic author was finding colleagues who were knowledgeable and generous enough with their time; to read drafts, offer comments, and help me and the profession to keep moving forwards. My 2 recent books and 10 of my last 11 papers acknowledge Dave for his editorial assistance. I share this with you because Dave's kind of selfless giving and collaboration is the lifeblood of the chiropractic profession.

When you look back at any of the great schools of philosophy in the history of the world, the best ideas developed through connections and rivalries. Innovation often happens when thought leaders, who are often friends, work together to combat challenges to the paradigm. In doing so, breakthroughs emerge. The chiropractic profession is involved, right now, in this type of innovative transformation. A small group of academics has been actively trying to steer the profession away from the traditional chiropractic paradigm and towards a biomedical paradigm. In the dynamic pushback against this, Dave was a central player. His efforts helped to pave the way for chiropractic's future.

Innovation, collaboration, and the development of chiropractic ideas have always occurred behind the scenes in letters, conversations, and personal connections. Letters from DD Palmer to BJ Palmer, written in 1902, include DD's first use of the term "sub-luxation," new techniques for chiropractic analysis, and rationales for not mixing Chiropractic with other methods. DD Palmer developed his ideas in conversation with dozens of his friends and students like OG Smith, TF Ratledge, Willard Carver, AP Davis, Sol Langworthy and especially BJ Palmer. In DD Palmer's many critiques of other chiropractic theories, he developed his ideas and established a unique chiropractic paradigm.

DD Palmer's paradigm emerged in the context of debate and innovation. In his final years, DD Palmer proposed that chiropractic is based on tone. Tone is the tissue's ability to bounce back to normal health, the real entity. The central chiropractic practice involved correction of the vertebral subluxation, which he defined as a dis-relationship between articulating surfaces of two vertebrae, whereby the open side of the joint was impinging upon neural structures. Vertebral subluxation led to abnormal function of the nerves, either too much or not enough functioning. He referred to such a state of tension or slack on the neuroskeleton, as dis-ease, which led to disease processes. In a letter written one month before he died, DD wrote, *"Chiropractic is the science (knowledge) of the principles which compose the scientific portion of Chiropractic. Chiropractic is divided into 3 grand divisions, the Science, the Art, and the Philosophy. The Art is subdivided into palpation, nerve-tracing and adjusting... Nerves are stretched; tension my boy causes 99 per cent of all diseases."*

Letters, articles, books, conversations, and teaching are how the profession evolves.

BJ Palmer's ability to support and challenge his students to become thought leaders was legendary. The most famous one was probably Shegetaro Morikubo. In 1907, his court case established that Chiropractic had a distinct philosophy, science, and art. Morikubo stated that he and BJ worked out the legal arguments for 6 months. The early authors of textbooks at the Palmer School of Chiropractic were BJ's students, friends, and collaborators such as Burich, Vedder, Firth, Craven, and Mabel Palmer, his wife. A decade after BJ published the first chiropractic Green Book in 1906, Craven collaborated with him, and they issued new editions of Volumes 1, 2, and 5, the philosophy texts. RW Stephenson's chiropractic textbook, published in 1927, was a homage to both BJ and Craven, his philosophy teacher. These early friendships and collaborations were the crucible through which the central ideas and practices of Chiropractic emerged.

BJ Palmer's chiropractic theories developed over 50 years. It would be difficult to count the many collaborators, students, and professional leaders he inspired. BJ's innovations included the normal complete cycle (1909), spinal X-ray analysis (1910), spinal cord pressures (1911), thermographic instrumentation (1924), along with myriad technique developments including the toggle adjustment and the upper cervical specific approach. He also continued to evolve the philosophical premises of chiropractic, well into his final years. BJ Palmer impacted 3 generations of chiropractors.

The most significant historical challenge to the chiropractic profession in the early 20th century was the Basic Science Laws. The medical lobby was stymied in its attempts to destroy the young profession in the courtroom, so it enacted laws across the United States requiring all health professionals to pass science exams written by professors at medical schools. New licences for chiropractors in some states dropped to zero for many years.

The profession met the challenge in 2 ways. School leaders that sought to align chiropractic with biomedicine increased their use of medical diagnostic textbooks in their curriculum and distanced the philosophy of chiropractic from clinical practice. Other thought leaders integrated contemporary scientific theories and textbooks into the chiropractic paradigm. The collaboration amongst these visionary chiropractors established a new level of academic rigor for the profession.

The 2 most innovative approaches were integrations of the works of AD Speransky and Hans Seyle. Speransky's book, *A Basis for the Theory of Medicine* was translated into English in 1935. In Speransky's theory of medicine, placing neural dysfunction on centre stage, chiropractors found empirical evidence for their central theories. BJ Palmer was quoting Speransky as early as 1938. One chiropractor, Arthur Heintze, travelled to Russia in 1936 to attend a lecture by Speransky. Heintze pioneered the concept of proprioception in chiropractic theory. He also inspired RJ Watkins and JR Verner to study Speransky.

Speranskian vertebral subluxation theories became central in the profession. From this perspective, the vertebral subluxation is a part of a global neurological and noxious phenomenon. The chiropractic adjustment disrupts the neuropathophysiological process. Chiropractors like Verner and RJ Watkins corresponded, collaborated, and inspired each other and many others. They integrated Seyle's stress theory into subluxation models as well. It is impossible to discuss modern vertebral subluxation theory without understanding how these pioneering chiropractors developed, researched, and modelled new approaches based on the leading science of their time.

Another crucible for the profession came in the 1970s when

the United States Department of Education acknowledged the Council on Chiropractic Education (CCE) as the sole accrediting body for chiropractic. The CCE was born from the biomedical side of the chiropractic spectrum, and its dominance of chiropractic education for the last 4 decades has impacted the profession in countless ways. One innovation that emerged from that crisis in chiropractic education came from collaborations and dialogue among chiropractors like Reggie Gold, Thom Gelardi, and their colleagues. They codified BJ Palmer's innovations from the 1930s through to the 1950s by distinguishing the importance of the analysis and correction of the vertebral subluxation in and of itself, for human health and wellbeing. Today we would add salutogenesis. Their movement inspired several chiropractic colleges worldwide and a generation of chiropractors.

In my collaborations I have attempted to honour this tradition of collegial dialogue, furthering and developing models of those who came before, and pushing the profession forwards. Mentors and colleagues I have worked with include David Koch, Ralph Boone, Dave Serio, Donald Epstein, Daniel Lemberger, Brian McAulay, Stevan Walton, Timothy Faulkner, Joseph Foley, Christopher Kent, Matthew McCoy, and Dave Russell. I've sought to demonstrate ways that the history of ideas in Chiropractic should be situated within a contextual time and place. Chiropractic developed alongside 20th century theoretical biology and integral theory, and has contributed to new ways of understanding physiology, health, wellness, and even consciousness.

My work with Dave was mutually collaborative. He was always thrilled to learn of my latest discoveries or insights and would integrate them into his writings. I have so many files saved in my computer with the initials "DR edits" appended to the title. I know many other thought leaders in the profession have similar files. Dave's contributions will be missed, but the spirit of intellectual support, growth, and collaboration will continue. Dave has been instrumental in pushing the profession forward. Chiropractic ideas are developing and evolving in dialogue within the profession's intellectual field.

Dr Russell was set to be the first president of the Scotland College of Chiropractic. He was involved in the launch of the school from its earliest days. Hopefully his life and works will inspire you, knowing that you are part of a grand tradition in this relatively young profession, only in its second century. You don't have to be a researcher or an author to model the attributes of excellence, collaboration, and professionalism that he embodied. Just do your work and do it well, with colleagues, in connection, and with the intent to document the best of Chiropractic and improve upon what has come before.

Wisdom #17

Marc Hudson DC

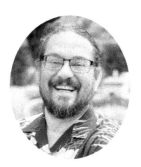

Marc Hudson has practiced on the beautiful island of Mallorca for 25 years. He is one of Europe's busiest chiropractors. He and his wife Lynn are the leaders of ChiroEurope: the heart and soul of the European vitalistic community. They were part of the small group that founded Barcelona Chiropractic College. For 20 years, they have coached chiropractors to massive success and happiness.

In addition to practicing, running seminars, involvement in Willow Life, and coaching, Marc and Lynn find time to be part of Life West's biannual India mission. On these missions, Marc organises DCs as they see thousands of patients. Lynn leads the daily meditation and gives health talks prior to care. She holds the world record for number of health talk attendees.

"WTF?"

The woman was thrusting a cushion towards me. On it lay a dead baby. At least, it looked like it was dead; nothing more than a limp, skeletal body. I tried to focus. The woman was telling me in Spanish that her baby had been born 9 months earlier and had been paralysed by the birth process. He spent his first 7 months in the ICU of the hospital before the medical doctors gave up and sent him home "to die with dignity".

The woman pushed the baby at me even more urgently as

I took a step backwards. Time slowed down and everything felt like it had gone into slow motion. Everything except the voice in my head which screamed: "Get that baby away from me!"

But the mother was insistent.

She and I were standing in the centre of the 5 basketball courts of the Gimnasio Roberto Duran, a massive sports complex in Panama City. It was hot, sticky and noisy. We were surrounded by thousands; organised chaos. I thought they were all watching me at this very moment.

I didn't know it then, but the decision to take the dying child from her would change the direction of my life forever.

It was 1998. I had come to Panama with a group of over 80 chiropractors for my first ever chiropractic mission. I had just started on a voyage of discovery. My journey to a time when I would fully embrace vitalistic chiropractic.

I came to Chiropractic through a sports injury. I broke my shoulder in a judo competition. When conventional medicine and physiotherapy failed to heal it after 6 months of treatment, I sought out a chiropractic intern at the local chiropractic school. After just a few visits, I had seemingly miraculous results. A few years later, my wife also had fantastic results with sciatica. I was looking for a change in my career and chiropractic seemed like a good choice.

I attended Parker University in Dallas. When I graduated, I saw Chiropractic as a biomechanical therapy and little more. We left Dallas and set up practice on a beautiful Spanish island in the Mediterranean.

After 2 years, I had a moderately successful biomechanical practice in what felt like paradise. My wife, Lynn, helped run the office. When viewed from the outside, my life looked successful.

Yet I was lost and felt completely fake. It was a horrible feeling to think I had spent so much time and energy, and taken on massive debt, to learn something that was not at all emotionally and energetically rewarding. I had no purpose or mission or drive other than job success. I knew there had to be more than this.

It was almost by accident that I discovered vitalistic chiropractic. After 2 years away from the States, we went back for a family vacation. I wanted to take advantage of that time to go to some chiropractic seminars and conferences. I chose one that I didn't know much about, but the schedule conveniently overlapped with our vacation.

It was at this seminar that I began to understand that chiropractic was so much more than they had taught me at school, so much more than what I was experiencing in my practice.

From the stage, I heard some of the legends of our profession. Dick Santo, Jim Sigafoose and Dr Sid Williams. I don't really remember what they said, but I was blown away by the energy in the room and the passion and purpose that was radiating out of everyone. I spoke to chiropractors around me in the audience who were practicing with such freedom and authenticity that I was blown away.

That weekend was a paradigm shift of epic proportions. When we returned to Spain, I was determined to make changes in my practice. And so my journey began.

It wasn't easy. We didn't have the internet then. I didn't know any subluxation based DCs. There was no community to support me in my journey. No ChiroEurope seminars, no coaching groups. We were isolated and alone. So, when I found out about the Panama mission trip that Jim Sigafoose and Dick Santo were leading, I jumped at the chance to go with them. I heard stories of previous Panama missions that added to my excitement. They spoke of chiropractors adjusting thousands, in overflowing stadiums. They spoke of witnessing chiropractic miracles during the days, and long nights of chiropractic philosophy.

That was how I came to be standing in the centre of a huge stadium, holding a dying baby. I was about to change his life story and also my own.

I had not come to Panama to adjust babies. In fact, I had never adjusted a baby in my life. I was trained to adjust adults with pain and injuries. Yes, I was transitioning to providing vitalistic care to my patients, but my journey was slow. I looked down at the lifeless child. I was frozen. I had no clue what to do. But then a moment of clarity came, and my shaking hands and trembling spirit were calmed. I heard a voice in my head give me clear and understandable instructions. They seem ridiculously simple now, and almost silly, but it was what I needed to hear: "Find the bump and push on the bump."

I woke from my dream state. "Find the bump..." That was easy enough to understand. I palpated his neck and he had what felt like the blunt end of a pencil sticking out on the left side of C1 (yes, I remember this clearly years later!). It felt like the pencil was trying to force its way out through the skin. "Push on the bump..." and without thinking, I did it.

It was gentle. Just a pinkie toggle. But it was fast and clean. I held my breath. The baby started flexing and extending his thoracic spine. It looked like a baby's version of the wave you see in Network. He was flopping around on the cushion. The mother let out a scream and there was pandemonium all around us. The stadium erupted. That baby was no longer paralysed. We were witnessing a chiropractic miracle.

Because I was one of the few DCs who spoke Spanish, the mission organisers moved me to different locations each day, so I didn't get to adjust the baby again on that trip. But his mother brought him back twice every day to get adjusted. Back at our hotel at night, I heard that each day that the mission continued, his body got a little stronger.

When I returned to Spain, I decided that I wanted my own practice to be as close to my Panama experience as it could possibly be. In my health classes, I started to talk about what had happened in Panama. Soon, the people coming to the practice shifted from sports injury/musculoskeletal problems to what I call really sick. Not "I feel bad," but about-to-die sick. It was for any and every imaginable type of problem. Things that would never have come up before. And the great thing was that we began to witness chiropractic miracles. Not just one or two, but almost as a normal occurrence.

My confidence in what was possible through Chiropractic grew stronger and stronger. And I was fortunate to have my wife at my side in this journey. I feel sorry for any chiropractor whose partner does not fully embrace the importance of what we do. My experience from coaching chiropractors over the last several years has shown me that a chiropractor's long-term success and happiness is influenced by just how much support their partner gives to them on their journey.

To succeed, chiropractors have to unlearn massive amounts, and replace that with congruent beliefs and learn to practice in a way that protects them energetically so that they can be the great healer they want to be. Together Lynn and I were being asked more and more to teach this to other chiropractors.

In 2004, I returned to Panama for another mission. This time I brought Lynn and our kids with me. I wanted them to experience what I had, all those years before. So much had happened since 1998. I was a full-blown vitalistic chiropractor. Our practice was the busiest vitalistic office, not merely in Spain, but anywhere in Europe. And this was despite being on a small island and despite doing no advertising or outside promotions of any kind. Our ChiroEurope community was spreading across Europe.

When I stepped into that same large stadium, it was just as hot and noisy. There were still thousands of people waiting to get adjusted, but I was a different chiropractor. I knew in every cell of my body just what Chiropractic is capable of achieving in this world. I began to adjust one patient after another, establishing a rhythm, letting go of my ego, and embracing the connection of my innate with their innate. I was lost in service, but my reverie was broken by a woman shouting. "It's him! It's him! It's him!" She was pointing at me. And then she began to point to a boy playing nearby. "It's him! It's him!"

It was the dying baby. He had grown into a strong, healthy, active child. And I can take no credit for that. He was dying from interference in his nervous system. When the interference was removed, his innate knew what to do to save his life.

Today is the 125th anniversary of the birthday of Chiropractic. Thank you DD. Thank you BJ. Thank you Sid Williams. Thank you River Ribley, Jim Sigafoose and Dick Santo. Thank you to ALL the giants whose shoulders we stand on. If we can help you gain that clarity and vision and focus, we are here for you. Love to all.

Zarak Bartley

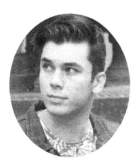

Zarak is currently a fourth-year student at the Barcelona College of Chiropractic and is an assistant coach for MLS seminars in Europe. He has a YouTube channel and podcast called Real Chiropractic Dynamics, in which he documents his chiropractic journey and interviews many different leaders of the profession.

Zarak's origins are unknown but it is believed he was formed in a lab by a team of scientists seeking to make the strongest chiropractor ever to exist, much like Captain America. He also tends to exaggerate when writing bios about himself.

Ask for what you need

When the group of remarkable people in charge of bringing the book you have in your hands into existence, asked me to contribute something I was very flattered. I am still a student, after all, I have yet to do anything significant in practice. Truthfully, I'm excited just to be around these guys. I would compare it to when Spider-Man (Holland, not Maguire) is excited and eager to learn just from being around the Avengers. He's not an Avenger yet but he is in training and just glad to be involved in some capacity. I can relate.

Then I wondered, if I haven't yet achieved anything significant in the profession, then what could I contribute that might be of some value to you? I hope that maybe this chapter can help a prospective student and also it might help the older guys to see what thoughts the students, the young blood are having regarding our amazing profession.

"What is unique about Chiropractic?" I've been asked. Well, many things.

I am sure the other contributors have given a multitude of unique messages and stories I always get inspired from hearing. For me, from a student's perspective, Chiropractic is the only profession in the world where I can call up the top performers in the game and pick their brains. It's quite an amazing opportunity.

We are so good to our students in this profession. I am lucky to have many mentors who have helped me with my growth and development along the way. To those of them reading this (you know who you are), I will always be grateful for everything you ever taught and I promise to pass it on to the next generation in years to come.

For the newcomers to the profession reading this, the key is that you need to be going to seminars. Seminars are where the best and brightest of our profession congregate to share ideas. You know the final battle in Avengers Endgame when all the superheroes come together? That's basically ChiroEurope. For me, anyway.

When you go to these seminars, don't be afraid to talk to the legends and ask questions. It can be intimidating to just go and sit opposite them and ask to pick their brain; I still even get nervous sometimes. But those are just nonsense thoughts and limiting beliefs in your head, trying to keep you in your comfort zone. The truth is that these badass chiropractors would be delighted to meet you and share with you, so put that nonsense chatter aside and go to talk to them. Some of the best pieces of advice I have ever been given took place during the coffee break or lunch at a seminar.

The whole reason I started my podcast was because there were so many times that I left the table thinking, "Damn, I wish I had taken notes or recorded that conversation!" But don't be needy and ask for stuff like a beggar; communicate with them authentically. I think that is the reason I am the only student in this book, because I always aim to communicate with authenticity and express my true opinion. I am not so good at being diplomatic or politically correct. It's not for everyone but amongst the right people, it's a breath of fresh air.

People resonate with authenticity. As I've said, seminars are where the best and most successful chiropractors congregate to share ideas. The anti-chiropractic forums where people complain about how hard it is to succeed, is where the losers congregate. Choose wisely.

Look for the chiropractors who have done what you would like to do, then emulate them. I much prefer to associate with those people who live a congruent life with the philosophy of Chiropractic and have achieved, or are working to achieve, objectives that resonate with me. Go and talk to the men and women you look up to. Listen to their stories. If you can forge these relationships, they are of extremely high quality and extremely sustainable because we are all working towards a common goal and can support one another.

We have an amazing opportunity to have fun and get great fulfilment from our work in Chiropractic. I think of the level of job satisfaction chiropractors have, compared to most people I know. What happens is that most people work a job they do not feel fulfilled by, that doesn't give them energy - in fact it takes a lot of energy from them and makes them miserable. So, when the weekend comes, they numb themselves by drinking copious amounts of alcohol in an attempt to shut down the mind and have a few brief moments of living without inhibition, before going back to work. They can't be present. So, because they can't be present, they can't receive any good energy anymore and then they have to poison themselves to shut their mind down, in order to feel present and feel good.

In other words, if there's no higher purpose to your life that serves to centre and ground you, then there is no real fulfilment. If there is no core reason why you are living your life, then every little problem is going to affect you. One of the main reasons I decided to become a chiropractor was seeing just how many of them do not want to retire. How many other jobs do you know where the person could easily retire but they just don't want to? They enjoy the hustle too much because they are engaged and have purpose.

Since Chiropractors get energy from helping people, we can feel we have a greater purpose in our community. We don't have to get bored with the work and that allows us to be present while we adjust. Let's appreciate the opportunity we have to enjoy ourselves while we make a living. I urge you to go and speak to the people excelling at it. I really think that if more students were exposed to this message, we would have a much stronger identity as a profession.

I refer back to my comment about authentic communication. What we offer is unique, yet we dilute it, because we aren't sure what we offer and we aren't sure of ourselves. If we don't know who we are and what we want, how can we possibly hope to convey that to the people in need of our services?

People who aren't sure in themselves tend to have that scarcity mindset and need to be accepted and acknowledged as the authority. You need to draw those boundaries between what we do and what other professions do and stand your ground. A lot of this stuff is entirely avoidable if you just stop trying to control everything and you trust the process and get some cool mentors. It's about hanging around people who are successful in practice, and doing what they say, rather than listening only to teachers in college who failed in practice, which can lead to failure teaching failure. Even if you pay to go to a seminar, the money you pay is enough to dissuade most of the losers from being there. The people who are there tend to have decent success in practice and you see what is possible.

People out there are not getting results, they aren't having success, they get frustrated about it, they don't even see the pathway to getting results in practice. They don't think, "Well if I learned the philosophy of my profession and showed that to the public, a few of them would probably like to come to me for help." They don't have an identity so a person might want a different approach to health that is above down inside out instead of the allopathic approach. But they just think: "Well I have to do something so I may as well learn some other remedies maybe sell some supplements and if I can make myself look like the other professions, maybe they will accept me." There certainly is a culture of that in Chiropractic.

People who don't see a pathway to a fun successful practice don't even take action to go down that path. They won't learn any philosophy or history and when they don't see immediate results in their adjusting, instead of practising the adjusting and mastering the art, they just go looking for something else to compensate. If they just understood, it's about asking what are the skills I need, what do I need to know, what worked for other chiropractors in the past and how do I explain to my patients how this is a different approach to looking after your health.

If they went down the path of developing those skills and educating themselves a bit on what makes us different, that would give them the confidence to at least start taking action. And if they started taking action, maybe they would get a few positive experiences which would encourage them to get into that upward spiral of getting more knowledge and putting that knowledge into action.

That's how you get into that positive cycle, find good mentors and educators and you'll develop that belief that we have something different and it really works. A lot of these guys just don't have good mentors, they become dissatisfied with the profession and they don't have anyone to guide them, to help them see things differently. Once you see what's possible and you get a few positive reference experiences of your own, it gives you much more confidence in the profession and an understanding of what we offer.

Why did Chiropractic come through all that oppression if we weren't doing something right in the first place? What changed? Did Chiropractic change or did we change?

We are unique in that we offer people something different, something they really need in these times. We can be deeply fulfilled by our work and (if we ask for it) the leaders of the profession are happy to show us the way.

Looking forward to growing with all of you on this journey.

Wisdom #18

FJ Schofield DC

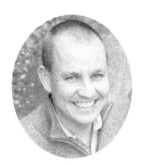

FJ is a second-generation chiropractor who grew up in Phoenix, Arizona. A keen sportsman, he attended Florida Atlantic University on a tennis scholarship and received a Palmer Rugby Scholarship, serving as Rugby Captain before graduating in 2009.

Prior to opening his own practice in West Bend, Wisconsin with his chiropractor wife, Korie, he worked for his father Fred Schofield DC which was an amazing apprenticeship. His absolute certainty and fine grounding enabled him to grow quickly. He and Korie now have 2 beautiful children and continue to grow their NUCCA practice.

Chase Your Joy

As a young boy I would wake up as soon as the sun was up and run outside to play basketball. I didn't do this for notoriety, acceptance or the possibility of future championship. No, I did it for the joy of playing. This went on for years. Nearly every day I would get up at around 5am and sometimes I was even able to drag my brother out to play with me.

Often, I would continue playing all day and would only stop when I was so thirsty or hungry my hands were shaking. At night I would beg my parents to let me keep playing in our driveway, under the streetlights.

I played because I loved to play. Of course, I played other

sports as well and was forced to play a musical instrument for a while, but nothing gave me the same joy as simply shooting a basketball.

My whole childhood, my father strongly encouraged me to play tennis. He and my mom were both short, so it would be hard to excel at basketball when I grew older, but he'd explain to me that I had a chance to be very good at tennis. I liked tennis and I enjoy competition but I never exploded out of bed in the early morning to play tennis.

However, I slowly started listening to my father and in 8th grade I decided to only play tennis, in an attempt to become very good and play professionally. It was a much more difficult sport for me to play and I didn't take to it as I had basketball.

I did enjoy it but a lot of that joy came from the belief that one day I would be great, rather than the joy of simply playing. There were many moments of extreme frustration and disappointment, because of my slow progress.

Throughout this whole experience, there was always a feeling in my gut, a feeling that I was forcing it. I was pushing hard right now, so one day it would be fun and great. When I was really good then it would be super-fun. When I was winning tournaments, then I would be happy.

I would, through a lot of hard work and frustration, become pretty good at tennis. I eventually played at Florida Atlantic University, earning an athletic scholarship, captaining my team in my junior and senior year. I was awarded the male student-athlete of the year award in my senior year and was acknowledged 3 times as being one of the best players in my conference.

But I was never going to be good enough to make a living

as a professional and play at Wimbledon. These were dreams that had been a big part of why I quit basketball and started playing tennis. I will never forget as I walked to my first class in Freshman year, passing the starting point guard and noticing he was much shorter than me. I instantly thought, "You mean I could have kept playing basketball and ended up here anyway?".

I have not picked up a racket in years but I still enjoy the occasional basketball shootaround. Would I have played in college had I kept playing basketball, I don't know and it doesn't matter. What does matter is the lesson. The lesson that our purpose and our path will always be revealed by having the courage to chase our joy. It doesn't mean you won't need to work hard and overcome adversity. It means that the work won't feel like work most of the time and the adversity will never make you consider quitting, because you love what you do.

I have learned my lesson and I am so grateful I had this experience. Now when I am faced with any decision in life, I always evaluate my feelings first and ask what truly brings me the most joy. I don't look at it logically or practically. I always look at it emotionally first. I believe we all have an innate intelligence that knows where we should go and what we should do and this internal guidance system speaks to us through gut feelings.

I had the choice of taking over my father's chiropractic practice or starting my own. His office is established and successful. It would have been much easier to take over his but my gut feeling urged me to start my own. So, I did.

When choosing the location for my practice, everyone was telling me to go to the Chicago area as it had the best reimbursement in the world and it would be much easier to build a successful practice in Chicago than it would in my wife's hometown of West Bend, Wisconsin. However, I chose West Bend because it felt right.

I decided to change the technique of my practice to upper cervical specific, because of an adjustment I had at a seminar in a chiropractor's office one time. It was just a feeling I had.

I decided to hire 2 associate chiropractor's, even though everyone told me I shouldn't. It was a gut feeling.

All these decisions and so many more, were all based on this lesson and I am so glad I've listened to my feelings. It has rewarded me in a level of success, happiness and fulfilment that I think few people ever know. Most people are stuck chasing someone else's dream and if you do that, you are only living for the end result. The money, the status; these rewards mean little if you don't love your day-to-day process.

I spend almost every day, all day, doing what I love to do. Now don't mistake what I am saying, all these decisions were implemented and executed with a lot of logic and practicality. But the initial decision was first guided by chasing my joy.

Practicality is so often disguised as fear, so we take the easier path or the path that is approved by our family and friends, because we are afraid. Afraid we might fail. The sooner you start listening to your inner voice, the sooner you will start moving towards a life of joy, fulfilment and yes, of course, success.

There will be tough times and there will still be doubt and frustration but when you have found your calling the highs will be euphoric and the day-to-day grind will not feel like such a grind. It will feel more like playing, because you had the courage and toughness to chase your joy.

Fred Schofield DC

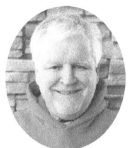

Since 1981, Fred and Susan Schofield have been dedicated to helping chiropractors, their spouses, staff and patients to break the barriers of mediocrity. Born in South Africa, Fred has a uniqueness, excitement, and intensity about him. He is truly One of a Kind.

Both player and coach, working in his office and coaching chiropractors one on one, he dedicates his time to enhancing planet Earth and the health of humanity through applying and understanding the Principles of ChiropracTic. Together with his wife, he co-founded Atlas Chiropractic Centre and Schofield Chiropractic Training, working worldwide.

Susan Schofield, a retired pharmacist now ChiropracTIC advocate, is considered a leading expert in Organizational Infrastructure and Management Technologies. Susan has designed and helped implement the procedures and protocols for million dollar, high-volume, patient-centred clinics.

It's game time!

"Everything is energy and that's all there is to it. Match the frequency of the reality you want and you cannot help but get that reality. It can be no other way. This is not philosophy. This is physics."
Albert Einstein

It was 1976 and I was playing professional rugby in Italy. I had injured my index finger, a compound fracture on my right hand and needed to come home for a third operation.

My father was a medical doctor and wine farmer. I knew nothing about Chiropractic except that a buddy I played rugby with was a chiropractor. I only knew the allopathic model (treat the symptom and chase the disease) and I had no idea that Chiropractic had a philosophy, a science or an art of healing from above down inside out. But I was about to find out.

I popped in for a pint at the renowned Capetown watering hole The Pig and Whistle and ran into a friend, Dr Steven Hillock, who I hadn't seen for years. We talked about my future and Dr Steven spoke of Palmer College of Chiropractic in America, where he had a scholarship to play rugby and had completed his chiropractic degree.

Dr Steven said, "You're going to become a chiropractor Freddy." I turned to another friend of mine, Tony Morse, and asked, "How do you know when it's time to make a life decision?" Tony told me, "Stop thinking so much and just do it."

I turned back to Dr Steven and said, "It looks like I'm going to America to become a chiropractor... and to play Rugby."

Fast forward to 1978, I was in a room listening to a world-famous chiropractor, Dr Bill Bahn (Muhammed Ali's chiropractor), lecturing on the science of the concussion of frequency, the inner game of health and life. I was fascinated. He said the inner game was all about alignment; alignment of the mind (iNNATE physiology) and the psychology. When all the cells in our body are in alignment (your cortex thots, your limbic system emotions and the neuromusculoskeletal system) we have balance between the internal atmosphere the external environment resulting in health!

I never knew there was an inner iNNATE game to health and life. It was a life-altering realisation to know that we all have an internal atmosphere and when we cultivate that internal physiology, then we stimulate, activate and motivate our internal resistance and immunity-activated from "above, down, inside, out."

Chiropractic principle 17 states:

"Every effect has a cause, and every cause has an effect." Sounds like my friend Sir Isaac Newton!

All biological systems have input and output or rather afferent sensory input and efferent sensory output; input equals output. You can't get out what you don't put in; for every action there is an equal and opposite reaction.

You are an energy management system. You stimulate, activate, motivate, and elevate your physiology through daily discipline in your personal life. What an awakening! POW. "Physiology of Winning," I was plugged in, turned on and tuned up!

The vortex had been stimulated, activated and motivated and now my physiology was elevated!

What time was it? Gametime!

Here I was at 25 years young, having gone through a quarter of my life without anybody ever talking to me about this Physiology of Winning, adjusting the inherent recuperative power within.

We must stay awake. We must stop sleeping our lives away. Now I was on fire with iNNATE GAME!

Work on the input, the output WiLL take care of itself.

It's the LAW of Health, Happiness and Prosperity.

Cause = Effect | Input = Output

I was fired up! Set the tone through the power of the adjustment.

Now came the tricky part. I had to figure out a system to activate my internal physiology on a daily basis. I had to trust the process. Your physiology is a self-healing, self-organising, self-directing, self-adapting organism (*The Tree of Knowledge*, by Maturana and Varela).

At all times (and for the last 6.2 billion years) our physiology has been adapting to our internal atmosphere and external environment. However, if there is interference to the sensory afferent input then it prevents the physiology from adapting, resulting in the output, symptoms and therefore Dis-Ease. High blood pressure is a symptom of tension on the circulatory system and not the cause of the tension. These are the effects, so stop treating the symptoms.

Once the interference to the sensory afferents is removed (through the adjustment) then BOOM, health is the outcome.

Your body's innate intelligence (the inherent recuperative power) has the database for healing; 500 million years of evolutionary stimulus sits in your brain stem.

Our reptilian brain knows how to heal a broken bone; just set the bone (alignment) and time will heal. Once we remove the sensory afferent subluxation through the adjustment, all else will follow.

Perhaps the human organism was designed as an energy-efficient organism controlled by the central nervous system (CNS), peripheral nervous system (PNS) and autonomic nervous system (ANS); a unique, magnificent, biological organism designed and driven by your vision, mission, and purpose. Set the tone and all else follows.

I am in this all the way!

Healing comes from the inside out and all else will follow.

Today I coach alongside my wife, my family and our team, together training over 25,000 chiropractors worldwide. We apply these situational and organisational tools (with science) to create the skills, knowledge, confidence, and clinical certainty in a clinical setting.

The major system of Chiropractic is to align the whole system – CNS, PNS, and ANS of your innate physiology. You are more than 7 systems; you ARE an innate Mind Energy, Vibration and Frequency field is everything.

Chiropractic is super, great and simple, but super-complex in application.

The 4 Ts you should work on:

1. Trauma: All traumas you have experienced in life – get your lifeline checked
2. Tension: Tension on your ANS. Locate the stress in your life, get your tension checked.
3. Toxicity: Wuji'nate your gut. Detoxification of your ANS. Do it, do it, do it now!
4. Tonicity: Tonicity of your sensory afferent system – get your spine in alignment

What you plan about, you bring about! Focus on your HEALTH.

For every cause there is an effect, therefore for every input there is an output.

Here I am at 65, still plugged in, turned on and tuned in. I have no symptoms.

What time is it?

It's Game Time!

Be still and sow and so it is!

I CAN, I WILL, I MUST, I AM!!

Wisdom #19

Travis Corcoran DC, ACP

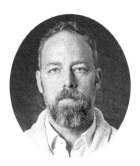

Dr Travis Corcoran is a proper philosopher and Liberal Arts enthusiast, who helps aspiring scholars both inside and outside the chiropractic profession to properly pursue the life of an autodidactic. Dr Corcoran is a proud graduate of Sherman's Academy of Chiropractic Philosophers and donates his time and finances regularly to colleges of Chiropractic, and principled chiropractic research.

His primary focus is to cultivate a strong sense of critical thinking in an effort to better manage and master one's emotions to better formulate constructive responses as opposed to emotional reactions.

How I have come to perceive the chiropractic landscape

In July 2004 I reluctantly visited a chiropractor in Chicago for the first time. A coworker practically dragged me to this appointment, like an uncooperative child. Hesitantly, I continued visiting the chiropractor. It only took 2 to 3 minutes to get checked and corrected when necessary, but my appointments were always a minimum of 20 minutes and upwards of an hour.

These appointments were lengthy due to the conversations between the chiropractor and myself about the different perspectives we both held concerning health and healing. My views on health included surgery when necessary, medicine, injections, exercise, and even massage. Her views on health and healing were radically different. She explained that she was going to check my spine for interference and then make a correction to restore neural integrity. Then, I would be able to optimally express my innate ability to adapt and subsequently heal myself in the time and manner that my own body deemed appropriate.

It was definitely a case of two different perspectives. Obviously, I discovered how incorrect I was, though that discussion is for later. For now, I do not want to focus on the differences in our knowledge. I want to focus on how she and I acquired our respective knowledge. This is called epistemology, in a word, "how we know what we know".

Dr Joseph Strauss begins *Chiropractic Philosophy* brilliantly; by discussing epistemology. What a great idea to discuss that first! He writes: *"Epistemology has been defined as the study of how we know what we know. It is the criteria by which truth is determined. In chiropractic philosophy, we use logic as the basis for determining truth."* (Strauss p.25)

That was the difference; epistemology was the difference between my knowledge and her knowledge. My knowledge was passive; it was from what my teachers, parents, or television told me. It was all social conformity, transferred authority, custom, and tradition. Ultimately, all these passive methods could be broken down into feelings. It felt good to trust my parents and teachers, and to believe that I was thinking for myself, when in fact I was not. Unbeknownst to me, I had a strong conviction bias and it gave me a false feeling of certainty. Ultimately, I did not understand the knowledge I possessed because I never questioned or properly evaluated it. However, my chiropractor's knowledge about health and healing was far from passive. It was active. She fully understood the knowledge she possessed.

Understanding is an active process that must be engaged. It is an investment of time and energy. I visited a chiropractor who did just that. One could acquire much knowledge by attending the right school. Understanding that knowledge is something else entirely. Lucky for me I visited a chiropractor who actually understood what she knew. Because of her knowledge and understanding, she became highly trained to detect and analyse subluxation.

I had earned a Bachelor of Science in Philosophy, so my knowledge and understanding meant I was highly trained to analyse and detect contradictions, fallacies, and errors of reason. Logic is an intense component of a university level philosophy programme, because logic is necessary to properly apply philosophy or wisdom, much like you need maths to apply the natural sciences; chemistry, biology, and physics. Just as mathematics has increasing levels of complexity, so does logic, starting with very simple pattern recognition, then Boolean logic, syllogisms, symbolic, sentential, and predicative logic.

During my appointments with the chiropractor, I honestly was not interested in understanding Chiropractic. I only wanted to prove her wrong, falsely believing this meant I would then be right or would achieve some imaginary intellectual victory. Despite my insincere mission and confrontational demeanor, she responded with perfect reasoning to my every query and objection.

Reflecting back on that time, I remain immensely grateful for how she responded. Her replies were always so elegant. With the perfect blend of confidence and grace, she answered each of my challenges to her profession and its philosophy. She was not in the least bit intimidated, because she stood so firmly and deeply rooted in her understanding of the principles and objectives of chiropractic.

Knowledge is very easy to acquire in this age of information. Knowledge is not power, but understanding it is. After 9 weeks of 3 sessions a week with her, I was sold. She had convinced me of the immense benefits that chiropractic offers, on the basis of reason and logic. She did not show me a single research study or article. It was pure reason that appealed to me.

At the end of those 2 months of appointments, chiropractic care was as true to me as the Pythagorean theorem is to a mathematician. So $a2 + b2 = c2$ is true to a mathematician because there are consistent geometric principles that are related to one another without contradiction. And that is why Chiropractic is true. Chiropractic is based upon related anatomical and physiological principles which are consistent with one another without contradiction.

My conviction was so strong, that 4 months after my first correction, I was seated in class for my first day of chiropractic school. However, I was surprised when I entered chiropractic school, and it still shocks me today. Why is there infighting in chiropractic? What is the dispute over? Mathematicians do not argue if the Pythagorean theorem is true or not.

The dilemma is very similar to the problem I had when I walked into that chiropractic office - knowledge without understanding. It is not as relevant whether that knowledge is correct or not. However, what is of tremendous relevance is the question, has the knowledge been evaluated? How was it evaluated? Was there any appeal to emotion? How can the knowledge be confirmed? This discussion is necessary, because ignoring the dilemma only allows the problem to continue. What happens when we do nothing about spinal degeneration? Does it get better? No. It only gets worse. Avoidance is not the answer.

To protect the integrity of this profession, there must be some degree of unity greater than exists currently. A profession divided, cannot protect itself any more than a divided army could protect its own castle. I would like to address or highlight this infighting, rather than avoid or neglect it. To do this I find it useful to first map out the perceived battlefield. This is best achieved by determining the borders or limits of the battlefield. What are the most extreme borders of the field, so to speak? Let us begin with a small pre-frame.

Life has at least two components; intelligence and matter, or the immaterial and the material. In the chiropractic profession, we have science to help us understand the material, and we have philosophy to help us understand the immaterial.

One extreme of our profession holds science and matter in highest regard. They have nearly a complete disregard for the philosophy or the immaterial component of life. The most extreme of the materialists have selectively discounted all immaterial components of life, except of course those that will fit into their parochial narrative, such as time or gravity.

The other extreme, views intelligence and philosophy in the highest regard. There is almost a complete indifference for science and matter. Inclusive to this most extreme perspective is the very dangerous worldview of solipsism, which easily leads to moral and scientific relativity.

When they speak among themselves, these 2 extreme groups are reinforcing their own confirmation biases. If they are presented with the other extreme's perspective, they react emotionally, which initiates a sympathetic stress response, fight or flight.

Science-matter extremists prefer fight and are typically antagonistic. They often aggressively demand to see the research (that only fits their narrative), discount accredited scientists and articles that contradict their scientific zealotry, labelling it pseudo-science, and default quickly to ad hominem attacks.

The other extreme prefers flight. They would like to withdraw and avoid conflict or neglect the pain of facing the issue, thereby allowing it to grow and fester. Often hiding a lack of courage or confidence by virtue-signalling how everything is "love". Other forms of professional escapism might include a feeble attempt to end a difficult discussion with, "everything happens for a reason", or "that is your or my truth."

There are brilliant and well-meaning people in both extremes. And they have a lot of suggestions about how to improve the chiropractic profession. However, everything they suggest is an outside-in solution, not an inside-out solution. The inside-out solution is quite simple. It begins in the individual mind of everyone in this profession. But that is not going to happen so long as we remain enslaved by our emotions.

One cannot control one's mind so long as an institution, individual, or ideology is eliciting emotional reactions. It is those external objects that are in control of one's mind, if one allows it. The only way to regain control of one's mind is to actively evaluate one's knowledge.

Knowledge without understanding is less than special, it can be destructive. Acquisition of knowledge is easy. Perhaps one can recite all 33 principles and quote their favourite chiropractic philosophers. Or another may be able to cite and reference multitudes of studies and research papers. However, does that mean that one understands either the principles or the research? One may be knowledgeable, but do they understand? That is the real question.

The early scholars and developers of our principles and chiropractic philosophy wished to collect more than knowledge; they wanted to understand. Why is one man sick while another man is healthy? They are both eating the same food and breathing the same air so why is it?

Thankfully, this profession has been gifted with many individuals who possess incredible understanding of the profession, its principles and objectives.

This quote by Dr Joseph Strauss on emotions and feelings, is profoundly concise: "[Feelings and emotions are] *one of the most common, and also one of the worst indicators of truth. ... There's nothing wrong with emotion. The human organism was given emotion for a purpose, but emotion is a responder to thought or action, not the precipitator of it. Each of us has different feelings that change from day to day, and in some cases, from moment to moment. This is far from an adequate method for establishing truth.*" (Strauss p.26, 27)

I would argue that emotion is an equally inadequate method of establishing our professional objectives, philosophy, and principles. And it is certainly one of the poorest methods for uniting this profession.

The chiropractic profession could be united, instead of divided. However, unity is just a slogan if we continue to react to one another emotionally. It is impossible to rally around turbulent and ever-changing emotions. But the stable, systematic, and reliable character of reason and logic is a worthy point of connection and unity. It is essential that individuals respond to each other with REASON and not react with EMOTION.

Monique Andrews MS, DC, DNM

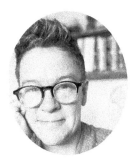

Monique Andrews, MS, DC, DNM is a chiropractor, neuroscientist and award-winning speaker who has been teaching about Chiropractic, the brain and the mind-body continuum for 20 years. She teaches internationally on topics such as the Neurophysiology of Subluxation, Neurodevelopment of the Paediatric Patient, Applied Polyvagal as Manual Neuroscience and the connection between Chiropractic and Consciousness. Affectionately known as Dr Mo, she is adored by students and docs for her ability to make even the most difficult concepts accessible.

She is the CEO of Dr Mo Knows, an interactive Science and Communication Mastery programme for chiropractors and chiropractic students. Last year Dr Mo co-founded The PRANA Foundation where she integrates western neuroscience with eastern spiritual practices to serve as a mentor facilitating masterminds and transformative retreats all over the world. Dr Mo's mission is to help human beings transform through mentorship, education, community and love. Few people possess the expertise, presence and wisdom to make a meaningful impact on humanity. Dr Mo is a rare gift.

Biohacking Consciousness

At any given moment there's a story playing in your head. It's like a never-ending movie that, were it not for sleep and moments of deep meditation, would be constantly streaming.

Just like a movie, it has vision and sound and emotion. You can think and dream, have memories and make plans. This eternal Netflix in your head is your stream of consciousness. And this never-ending movie, your stream of consciousness, is what makes you uniquely human. It has been argued that without it, life would have no meaning. Without our ability to reflect on self, on others, on our life, our lives would be meaningless.

So, if it's that important, why do we understand so little about it? It turns out that consciousness is probably the most complex construct in the known universe. In fact, it has been referred to as the "hard problem of science" and scientists pretty much stayed away from trying to understand it until the early 1990s when Francis Crick (yes that Francis Crick) published a paper titled, "Towards a neurobiological theory of consciousness".[7] The paper sparked a new curiosity and willingness to delve into the hard problem of science.

Fast forward to the present day and hundreds of scientists have spent thousands of hours uncovering a deeper understanding of consciousness. Now there are 2 prevailing theories. One has your brain as the storehouse of consciousness. In essence, your brain matter creates your consciousness and without your brain, consciousness wouldn't exist. In the second theory, your brain is merely a conduit with consciousness in

---

7 Crick F and Koch C (1990) *Towards a neurobiological theory of consciousness.* Seminars in the Neurosciences 2: 263–275

the field. This theory states that consciousness is outside of us and the brain is merely interpreting, transmitting, as it were, the field around us. So, take your eyes. They do not see, they are merely conduits for the visual information to enter and then be processed by the brain.

For the sake of this discussion, we'll put aside that argument and accept that either way, the brain is involved, somehow. Whether the brain creates consciousness or merely transmits it from the field, there have to be some specific areas of the brain that are doing the creating or transmitting.

The question then is this: where does consciousness reside? Neuroscience research is pointing to a few particular areas. Dr Richie Davidson did some of the early work into the neurobiology of consciousness at the University of Wisconsin in the 1990s. The landmark research supported the theory that the mind, both conscious and unconscious, was a function of the nervous system and specifically the brain. Of even greater significance are the particular areas within the brain that have been attributed to being the seat of conscious experience.

Over the last 3 decades neuroscientists have been able to pinpoint a proposed anatomy of consciousness. Through advancements in neuroimaging, researchers have been able to show structural and functional evidence of neuroplastic changes in response to the human experience. The brain areas showing the greatest evidence of change are the prefrontal cortex, cingulate cortex and insula. The brain changes observed in experienced meditators are so great that they found that 20 experienced practitioners of one type of Buddhist meditation had a greater volume of brain tissue in the prefrontal cortex and insula than a control group![8]

This is where the story gets interesting for the chiropractor. It turns out that the areas that are involved in consciousness are the same areas most impacted by the chiropractic adjustment! Chiropractic studies in neuroscience have elucidated several central nervous system sites that evidence change when adjustments are made to the spine. Electrophysiological, metabolic and fMRI studies all point to some very specific and similar brain areas.

Dr Heidi Haavik's electrophysiology studies clearly demonstrate that the prefrontal cortex is one of the primary areas influenced by chiropractic adjustment. The New Zealand team used Electroencephalograph (EEG) to evaluate the impact of spinal adjustments on electrical brain activity. They demonstrated *"...solid scientific evidence that adjusting the spine changes the way the prefrontal cortex of the brain is processing information"*.[9]

Dr. Takeshi Ogura's metabolic studies mirror these findings in the prefrontal cortex and other consciousness rich areas. This team used positron emission tomography (PET) to assess glucose metabolism in the brain pre-and-post chiropractic adjustment. The research demonstrated changes in metabolic activity post adjustment in a number of areas including the prefrontal cortex, anterior cingulate cortex, temporal cortex, visual cortex and cerebellum.[10]

---

8 Fox et al. *Is meditation associated with altered brain structure? A systematic review and meta-analysis of morphometric neuroimaging in meditation practitioners* May 2014 Neuroscience & Biobehavioral Reviews 43
9 Lelic et al. *Manipulation of Dysfunctional Spinal Joints Affects Sensorimotor Integration in the Prefrontal Cortex: A Brain Source Localization Study* January 2016 Neural Plasticity 2016(8)
10 Ogura et al. *Cerebral metabolic changes in men after chiropractic spinal manipulation for neck pain* Ogura et al (2011). Alternative therapies in health and medicine. 17. 12-7

Functional MRI studies evaluating functional connectivity between brain areas also support the premise that chiropractic adjustment impacts centres of consciousness. One award winning study that investigated changes in functional connectivity between brain regions that process and modulate the pain experience posits *"... it is reasonable to assume that the underlying therapeutic effect of manual therapy is likely to include an higher cortical component."*[11]

Across all of these studies, one area in particular was commonly found to be of significance and it didn't matter how they were evaluating the brain. Whether it's EEG, PET or fMRI, when studying the impact of a spinal adjustment to correct vertebral subluxation, all of these researchers found the same underlying area involved; the prefrontal cortex.

The prefrontal cortex is deemed to be responsible for executive function, including things like cognitive function, working memory, critical thought, planning, goal setting, impulse interpreting and understanding the thoughts and mental states of ourselves and others. It becomes most active when you think about yourself and even more so if those thoughts are emotionally charged.

The prefrontal cortex also has the largest cortical component of the human brain and is the latest of any species to develop. In fact, it continues to develop until approximately 25 years of age. This could maybe explain the impulse control behaviour we exhibited as teenagers! I would argue that it is the frontal cortex that makes us uniquely human and that without it, life would hold no value. It is responsible for our ability to

---

11 Gay et al *Immediate changes after manual therapy in resting-state functional connectivity as measured by functional magnetic resonance imaging in participants with induced low back pain.* October 2014 Journal of Manipulative and Physiological Therapeutics 37(9)

interpret what we hear and read and write, paint masterpieces, build cathedrals, fall in love...

There was one other significant commonality across these studies; they all demonstrated that when we adjust the spine, we change the brain. Now if the brain is the primary orchestra conductor for every cell, organ and tissue in the human body, and neuroscience proves that we are impacting the brain with the chiropractic adjustment, then why aren't more people under chiropractic care?

Maybe, just maybe, it's because not enough of us are sharing that message. When we adjust the spine, we change the brain and not in a random fashion; and as we now know, not in a random place. We are impacting the prefrontal cortex and the insula, the areas of the brain responsible for our ability to sense, emote and interact with our internal and external world. The areas of the brain responsible for making us uniquely human, the areas responsible for our ability to experience the vast richness that we call life!

I once heard Donny Epstein say, *"We are not adjusting the spine, we are adjusting destiny."* I couldn't agree more. We live our entire lives through our nervous system. Above Down Inside Out. The research shows that Chiropractic creates positive changes in the brain in the areas that are responsible for human consciousness. That's the closest evidence I've seen for uniting the physical with the spiritual. Never before have we been offered a deeper understanding of our chiropractic purpose. I don't need a better argument for Chiropractic. Do you?

Change someone's brain and you change the life. It's as simple as that!

Wisdom #20

Gilles A. LaMarche BSc, DC

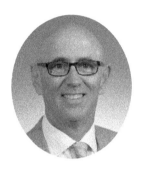

Giles is a Chiropractor, educator, passionate healer, accomplished author, professional speaker, and inspiring certified personal development/executive coach. He found his calling as a healer when at the age of 12 he was taken to a chiropractor after years spent as an "unwell" child. This would change the course of his life.

Giles is the author of 13 books and numerous articles, and has served as Vice President of University Advancement at Life University. He is also a member of The ASRF Research Review Panel and has appointments to numerous committees and boards in Cobb County.

The power of purpose and persistence

What a fantastic time to be alive, and what a fantastic time in history to be a chiropractor. Does this hold true for you or are you more likely to say, "Most of the time I don't have much fun, and the rest of the time I don't have any fun at all." Talented people are often prevented from fully participating in this game called life, due to fear, lack of confidence or simply lack of action. I share this information to inspire you to attain success, a success that perhaps until now, you had only imagined. My mission is to give you the insights and tools to create your ideal life and your ideal practice, so that no matter what obstacles, you have the ability to surmount them.

Confident, self-actualising people have a sense of purpose. They believe that they are important and that they matter. The confident individual understands that attitude originates within. Be aware of what you're good at, seek your special gifts and abilities. Success and satisfaction are simply rewards for sharing your special gifts with those who cross your path, making a difference. Yes, such endeavours require commitment. If you are willing to commit to what you truly value and believe, invest time in developing new strategies for your life and for your practice. Each part of you, physical, mental, and emotional must be aligned to win this game of life. The payoff for your commitment will be the accomplishment of your burning desire, leading you to a level greater than motivation, called purpose. Don't let the future be that time when you wish that you had done what you are not doing now.

Have you ever wondered how Chiropractic has survived constant attacks over the past 125 years, how chiropractors have thrived through years of persecution by members of the establishment? The answer is quite simple. It is the power of purpose and persistence; having faith, confidence and belief in the product, services and ideas of Chiropractic. It is staying steadfast in the understanding that truth always prevails.

DD Palmer stated, *"The science of Chiropractic has modified our views concerning life, death, health, and disease. We no longer believe that disease is an entity, something foreign to the body, which may enter from without, and with which we have to grasp, struggle, fight and conquer, or submit and succumb to its ravages. Disease is a disturbed condition, not a thing of enmity. Disease is an abnormal performance of certain functions; the abnormal activity has its causes."*

The science of chiropractic emphasizes the relationship between structure, primarily of the spinal column and the nervous system, and how that relationship affects function and health. Implicit within this statement is the significance of the nervous system to health and the effect of the subluxation complex upon the nervous system, and therefore, the entire body. Chiropractic relies on its major premise, that universal intelligence is in all matter and continually gives to it all its properties and actions, thus maintaining it in existence.

The expression of intelligence through matter is the chiropractic meaning of life. It is my belief that these concepts must be well understood by the chiropractor and shared with the public. As a profession, we have done a poor job in communicating who we are and the value we bring humanity. Not only have we failed to gain important cultural authority, often the mention of Chiropractic provides negative brand equity. And that, in my opinion, is due to the individual chiropractors' unwillingness or inability to teach the public about Chiropractic.

How many people stop because too few say, "GO"? Chiropractors and chiropractic students are a special breed of people with an inner ability to imagine, to envision, to be enraptured by the unseen, all hazards and hardships notwithstanding. How glad I am that certain chiropractic visionaries like Drs BJ Palmer, Jim Parker, Sid Williams, refused to listen to the short-sighted doomsayers who only saw as far as the first obstacle, and that present leaders like Drs Rob Scott, Ross MacDonald, Heidi Haavik, Stephanie Sullivan and so many more, remain steadfast, leading with authority, that Chiropractic is the best kept secret in healthcare. We must produce the research to support the paradigm and deliver this message to the sick and suffering. Secret no more, it is time isn't it?

Imagine where the world would be if Edison had given up on the light bulb when all his helpers doubted "the thing" would work; if Michelangelo had, faced with so many put-downs, stopped pounding and painting; if Steve Jobs had chosen to back off instead of persevering. The world is filled with people who quit trying, it is also filled with people who discovered the power of purpose and persistence, took concerted congruent action and accomplished what many said was impossible. The famous 18th century philosopher Schopenhauer stated that every great idea goes through 3 phases. First it is ridiculed, then it is violently opposed, and thirdly it is accepted as self-evident. When speaking to groups of chiropractic students, assistants and chiropractors, I often ask the question, based on Schopenhauer's assertion: "Where is Chiropractic now?" Most of the time, I receive a resounding "phase 1" or "phase 2" as the answer. That is no doubt defensive in nature and is only partially true. Many see chiropractic in phase 3; self-evident. Certainly, you do, and so do all people who have experienced the benefit of chiropractic care.

Chiropractic is at a major crossroads and in my opinion, we must unite as a profession under a common banner:

"The nervous system is the controlling system of the body and is adversely affected by spinal subluxation. Chiropractic improves and restores spinal function, leading to optimal brain function, neurological integrity and optimal health potential."

Under this banner, Chiropractic will thrive, people will experience better health and positive social change will occur. We must persevere with purpose as we face adversity. If

Chiropractic had no perceived value in the eyes of the masses, there would be no one opposing what we do as chiropractors. What you do matters. The power of purpose and persistence has kept Chiropractic alive, yet we need more of our colleagues to fuel this power of purpose and persistence. Chiropractic needs you to play full out, to be willing to tell the truth about who you are and what you do. If everyone knew what you know to be true about Chiropractic, they would all want to receive chiropractic care for life.

The ancient philosopher Patanjali was once asked: "Why is having a purpose for your life so important?"

His response was very clear: "*Because purpose inspires you. And when you are inspired by some grand purpose, your thoughts break their bonds, your mind transcends limitations, your consciousness expands in every direction, dormant forces faculties and talents come alive, and you discover yourself to be a greater person by far than you ever dreamt possible.*"

Do you think that life is meaningless, and that your existence is unremarkable? If so, this does not have to be your story. You can change it by writing a new story with purpose. A life of significance is built on the foundation of true purpose. Every morning when you wake, you're given a blank canvas, and the opportunity to create what will be displayed on that canvas. Who will you be and what will you do during those 1440 minutes of every 24 hours of your life? If you want to live a life of significance, it is imperative that you embrace the responsibility for finding your purpose and being the authentic author of your life. If you are willing to embrace responsibility to write your story, continue reading as I offer you tips and strategies for creating a purposeful life.

Life University was founded on the philosophy of the Lasting Purpose; to give, to do, to love, to serve from your own abundance, with no expectation of return. While understanding and living this philosophy gives one strength and direction, it is within your power to make your life a great story, one guided by your unique purpose. To live a life of purpose and significance, all you must do is make a difference to the lives of others wherever you are, in whatever role you play, in whatever capacity you can, with whatever you have, moment by moment, day by day. Doesn't sound very complicated does it? So, where do you start?

My mentors taught me that the starting point for all significance is purpose and a willingness to be fully committed. Life really isn't about sitting on the sidelines, it's about being fully engaged, enjoying the present moment, and being intentional. That calls for action, not excuses. Though not everything you face can be changed, and no past experience can be rewound, nothing can be changed until you face it. Leadership expert John C Maxwell has said, *"Being passive may feel safe. If you do nothing, nothing can go wrong. But while inaction cannot fail, it cannot succeed either. We can wait, and hope, and wish, but if we do, we miss these stories our lives could be. We cannot allow our fears and questions to keep us from seeking our purpose."*

If you want to live a life of purpose and significance, don't wait until you get good before you start, start now so you become great. You start so you can improve. You've probably heard the phrase "practice makes perfect". I don't believe that to be true. My experience has been that "practice makes improvement". I invite you to start thinking now, so you can begin to clearly define your purpose and improve in the direction you want.

When you say I'll do this, you unleash tremendous power within yourself, and that leads to commitment. While trying is filled with good intentions, doing is the result of committed action. A beautiful story will emerge for you when you are intentional. You will find yourself by discovering your purposeful path of significance by serving others. The people you help will develop greater significance for their life, and the legacy of reciprocity and service will live on. What small act of kindness could you initiate today? Could you choose to smile more, could you choose to greet people with more kindness, could you choose to say hello to everyone you meet, and give a heartfelt thank you to those who serve you? The answer to each of these questions is quite simple isn't it? Of course, you could. But will you? All it takes is one little step to begin the process, and that is where significance will be discovered and experienced.

In his book, *"The Purpose Driven Life"*, Rick Warren wrote, *"Humans are made to have meaning. Without purpose, life is meaningless. A meaningless life is a life without hope or significance. This is a profound statement and one that everyone should spend time pondering. God gives purpose. Purpose gives meaning. Meaning gives hope and significance. There is awesome truth contained within that logic."*

What thoughts do you wake up to in the morning? What thoughts drive your day, and what thoughts do you fall asleep to every night? I encourage you to ponder these questions and discover your answers. If the thoughts that govern your life are not allowing you to create the life you want, then it's time to insert new thoughts, thoughts of love, kindness, service and well-being. Start being kind to yourself and others, become familiar with your talents and your qualities, and embrace the beautiful you that resides within. When you do, your purpose will start emerging and it will become your rudder. Your purpose will give you direction and keep you on the right path even during tumultuous moments. People with purpose can keep their heads held high even during the most difficult of times. *"Your why is fuel for your strengths. And your strengths are the way to fulfil your why."* John C Maxwell.

If you have not yet discovered your why, your purpose, the first question you must ask yourself is, "How can I add value to others?" I encourage you to spend time in silence listening for the answer to that question. When you listen, you will receive multiple answers. Then start implementing the answers you receive. The Life University campus has multiple areas where you can sit in silence, enjoy nature, and ponder; from the Lasting Purpose pool to Lyceum Park, from the Tree House to the 19th century village path.

Here are some other questions you can ask yourself to get clarity and set you on the path to discovering and living your purpose:

What do I cry about?

What disturbs me?

What inflicts emotional pain?

What causes me so much discomfort that I'm motivated to take action and do something to bring healing to that situation?

What makes me happy?

What puts a bounce in my step?

What makes me jump for joy or spontaneously break into song?

What feeds my passion, what feeds my soul?

What do I dream about?

What could I do on a larger scale?

Yes, there are many questions. The quality of your life will depend on the quality of the questions you're willing to ask yourself and answer. Please take time to ask yourself these questions, discover your unique answers and create a plan to live them. You matter and you are significant.

Ralph Waldo Emerson said, *"The purpose of life is not to be happy. It is to be useful, to be honourable, to be compassionate, to have it make some difference that you have lived and lived well."*

I have a dream. A dream that within this decade, Chiropractic will be at the forefront of the health and wellness paradigm. To make this happen it is imperative that every chiropractor on the planet experiences, through the power of purpose and persistence, the success that she/he deserves, and that future chiropractors be attracted to this wonderful healing profession.

Sunlight focused on a magnifying glass can start a fire. The conditions, however, must be just right. If the magnifying glass is held too far from the surface, the rays are diffused and won't generate enough heat to make the fire. When you heat water to 100°C it begins to boil. If the temperature only reaches 99°C, water does not boil. An airplane has to attain a certain ground speed before taking flight. Any less speed does not produce flight.

Some doctors expend enormous amounts of energy trying to become successful. They seem to do almost everything correctly. They go through all the right motions, still success seems to elude them. Others appear to go through the same motions and are awash with abundance. What is the difference? To manifest and achieve abundance, you must achieve congruence; a condition where all parts of you are in alignment. The three key parts that must align are desire, belief, and self-acceptance. Desire, you must want it. Belief, you must believe that you can build and enjoy the practice of your dreams. Self-acceptance, you must believe that you deserve the success you seek. If one of these elements is out of alignment, your energy and focus diffuse. Congruency demands that all 3 engines be fired up to launch you forward. Every part of you must buy in – heart, mind and soul. I had the privilege and honour of being mentored by Dr James W Parker. He always reminded people that a thought and action equals a feeling. If you know what feeling you want to experience most of the time (such as success), you must think successful thoughts and perform success-oriented actions and you surely will achieve success. Success in Chiropractic is within your reach. Chiropractic shows you and, as such, you have everything it takes to successfully help thousands of patients discover outdoor health. It is time for you to prepare your mind and your heart, and to clarify and envision what you truly want for your life. By doing so, you will say yes to chiropractic success.

Chiropractors have fought a hard and diligent battle to be heard, yet chiropractic remains the best kept secret in healthcare today. I encourage all of you to participate in a paradigm and help every chiropractor share this message of hope with the world.

Let's choose to teach the message wherever we are, be proud to be a member of the greatest healing profession known to humankind, be proud to be a chiropractor.

Rebecca Vickery DC

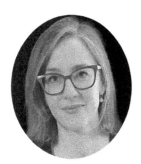

Rebecca Vickery graduated from RMIT in her native Australia and has now practised in the UK for over 20 years. She runs a family chiropractic practice in Edinburgh Scotland and together with her husband Ross she founded 'The Edinburgh Lectures' in 2006, an annual conference designed to educate and inspire Chiropractors and their teams. As a mother of three active children, Rebecca believes they are testament to how being a Chiropractor extends beyond your office walls.

What Chiropractic means to me

I don't remember my first adjustment, but apparently it was life changing. I was the screaming baby who settled, and for whatever reason was put on a path. The first adjustment that I do remember came several years later and fascinated me in a way I couldn't really describe. Today, after 20 years in practice, Chiropractic has continued to both fascinate and frustrate me. It has inspired me and disheartened me. There have been days when I can sincerely say I have the best job in the world, and others when I wish I was an accountant, so things were a bit more black-and-white.

Chiropractic has taken me around the globe and it has introduced me to the most interesting people in the world, as friends, colleagues, and those who have presented on my bench. It has made me doubt myself, while never questioning the importance of it, and its philosophy has given me a unique and valuable perspective on the world. And while I am proud to call myself a chiropractor, I have not always found it easy. Perhaps this was most prevalent when I was juggling part time practice with 3 small children. I spent every waking moment giving myself a hard time because I didn't think I worked enough hours, I didn't adjust enough people and worse still, that I wasn't the mother I imagined I should be. But during that time here is what I learned.

There is no such thing as a part-time chiropractor. Chiropractic is the filter through which you view the world. It is far more difficult to discuss it at the school gates than it is when you have a patient face down on the bench. And it cannot be switched off at the end of the day, particularly when you are raising a family. Being a chiropractor is exactly that, it is a state of being.

The quality of the chiropractor cannot be determined by the number of patient visits or the number of hours worked. To quote BJ Palmer, *"You never know how far reaching something you think say or do today will affect the lives of millions tomorrow"*. I know with absolute certainty that every person I put my hands on can benefit from chiropractic care. I also know that when you trust in the premise of the Big Idea, it is impossible to have a small practice.

Just last week I received a lovely compliment from a patient. She had said that her son-in-law (whom I had never met) had wanted to thank me. After a conversation some months earlier during an adjustment with his mother-in-law, I had suggested he should try Chiropractic. I have never met him and I don't know his chiropractor, but apparently it has been life changing.

Wisdom #21

Martin Rosen DC, CSCP, CSPP

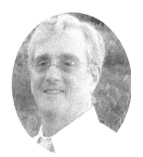

Martin graduated from Life Chiropractic College in 1981 and practices in Massachusetts, USA with his wife and daughter. He is the President Emeritus of SOTO-USA, chairman of their paediatric committee and the past president of the SORSI research committee.

Martin has produced numerous magazine articles, research papers, educational videos and technique manuals. His latest book, 2nd Edition of Pediatric Chiropractic Care is in its 3rd printing. He also serves as a post graduate instructor for several chiropractic colleges and is an international speaker and guest lecturer with his own lecture series.

A singular journey

I am writing this in a time that none of us would have thought possible. Our world is ensconced in a pandemic. As a chiropractor, and one who believes in a salutogenic model of healthcare, this is a philosophical and ethical conundrum. It is a perfect storm for the medical model of healthcare to perpetuate its preeminent position in the minds of the people of the world. Once again, we are dealing with an ambulance in the valley methodology (*The Ambulance Down in the Valley*, by Joseph Malins 1895) and not taking into account more encompassing and most likely more efficient preventative strategies.

Understanding the concept that health truly comes from

within, and manifesting that in your daily activities is something that we as chiropractors have been saying since the inception of our profession. Throughout my lifetime, both personally and professionally, I have always had a sense that my body had the ability to adapt and heal, given the proper materials, circumstances and personal responsibility to take care of it as best as I could. An outside in approach never really made sense to me. It always felt more like a way to patch things up, after I had pushed past my limits beyond the point where my body was able to adapt.

We now live in a time where these 2 philosophical constructs are meeting, head-on. We as chiropractors, as always, have an opportunity to offer a more rational, less fear-based approach to dealing with the world, that needs a more effective, efficient and rational way to maintain its health, approach disease and adapt to our ever-changing environment. It is times like these that test our mettle. Who are you, what do you stand for, where is your place in this world and what are you willing to do? These are questions that not only we as chiropractors, but as human beings often ask ourselves; and struggle with. Finding our place, making our mark, contributing to society; how we do this is a reflection of our ability to look inside, ask ourselves the difficult questions and be honest with our answers.

Once we have answered these questions, and yes, I understand that answers change and vary as we grow and change, the next step is to find the strength, trust and compassion to "walk the talk." I feel one of the most effective ways to do this is to try to approach this process without judgment of others. Understanding that we each have our own process does not in any way negate or weaken your individual process, position or beliefs. Throughout my life, and particularly my professional career as a chiropractor, I have often met opposition to the tenets of my belief system. What has served me during these times is 2 main things: the trust that my internal process that has brought me to where I am at that point in time has been as true and insightful as possible, and that while I'm willing to listen to the opinions of others, I am not attached to their personal view of me. What this means is that I do not feel the need to change or accept what either of us are saying simply to make them happy or have them approve of me.

Another driving force that I have gleaned from watching others who have lived rewarding and fulfilling lives, is to always have an end game that is bigger than yourself. It is my experience that the bigger the purpose for your actions, the easier it is to stay true to your beliefs and to stay on course regardless of the opposing forces you face along the way. Many years ago, I read an essay titled *"How to Walk the Path of Life"*. What moved me in this essay was the realisation that we will frequently get frustrated, sometimes even broken, by obstacles in our life. These obstacles will never stop coming, and instead of blaming their presence or their actions for our failures, often the best way to approach these obstacles is simply to find our own way around them or between them. We must be much more concerned about finding our own path, rather than focusing on moving all those obstacles we think are blocking our path, out of our way. We must keep walking our path without worrying about those who try to block our way.

I have found that trying to convince, cajole, prove your point, or move someone over to your side, wastes much of your precious time, energy and focus. It is often a futile task; to try and convince people to follow your way or move them from your path. Staying true to, and focused on, your objectives and finding a more compassionate and less abrasive way around the situation once you realise that their change has to come from inside them, will save you time, energy and strength. So you will be better able to continue on your way, facilitate your growth, allow for your transitions and realise your true purpose.

The question I have often asked myself and my students is, "What drives your practice and your life?" There are hierarchies from which we move forward in our lives. These are often based on a variety of circumstances and situations. Not unlike Maslow's hierarchies, there is a need to experience and process the previous level, before ascending to the next. For the purpose of this essay, I have defined them into 3 driving forces: ego, growth and mindfulness. When discussing or evaluating these parameters it is important not to judge where you are, but to be aware that movement forward is the driving force.

As these relate to your practice and life, the ego phase is akin to a survival level where you are striving to make money to live, create a level of success that will satisfy you and give you the ability to move forward and find prestige or acceptance (hopefully of yourself, not based on others' perception). The growth phase can often be a time of pure enjoyment and immersion in the process, seeing your goals and aspirations come to fruition and knowing that you are making a difference. This phase is often the longest of the 3 because it fills so many of your needs, emotionally, materialistically and neurologically, increasing the constant flow of endorphins as goals are met and actualised.

Finally, the state of mindfulness is a place where you can

truly encompass the ideology of the greater purpose that was your motivating factor. Service for the sake of service, compassion, and ultimately the choice to do what you want and be who you are without the encumbrances associated with the previous 2 phases.

The success of this process is dependent on you making conscious decisions, following through with them, not blaming others for your failures, accepting your failures and moving on, staying true to your inner voice and moral and ethical compass. Not an easy task and I can guarantee there will be many ups and downs in this process. But time, patience and consistency will be effective tools you can count on to make your way through.

What I love about Chiropractic is that it is not only a profession, but a philosophical construct that can be a guide for you throughout life. The ideology that there is an internal mechanism that is ever-present, and always working to create balance in your best interest is, especially in challenging times, a great comfort. Knowing that, given the right materials, opportunity, and unimpeded by external interference, this process knows what is right for you to maintain homeostasis at all times. This internal force is also connected to a greater universal consciousness that maintains things in existence. The realisation and acceptance of the existence of these two collaborative forces can help you create an inner strength that can empower your life and all of those whose lives you come into contact with.

I have built my practice on the premise that if I can locate and facilitate the correction of subluxations in the individual to the absolute best of my ability, the healing process within them will unfold to its greatest potential. While Chiropractic encompasses an art, science and philosophy, as a practitioner I have always believed that the art is the strongest and most important part of the triad. If you have the ability to perform the adjustment at the highest level possible, the outcome will speak for itself. Philosophy will open the door to those who gravitate to your thought process, science will secure the efficacy of the modality you purport, but the art, the delivering of the adjustment, will be the empirical parameter by which you and your practice will ultimately be judged.

Your practice is a reflection of your life because it is an integral part of who you are, what you believe and how you show up in the world. This relationship is no different to any of your personal relationships. It brings you joy, sadness, confusion, frustration, satisfaction, respect, abundance, struggle, reverence, respect, humility and love. To succeed, the relationship with yourself must also be one of compassion, honesty, reflection, respect, acceptance and love. I have been in practice for 38 years and have had the honour of taking care of 3 generations of family members. This has been a sacred trust for me and even in the most difficult of times, the ideology and art of Chiropractic has been both a beacon and a lifeboat for me and my family.

Your journey will be singular for you. It may be harder, it may be easier, it may have a different ending to mine, but understand it will be your choice to make the most of it, regardless of the circumstances, challenges or obstacles you encounter.

Ana Echeveste DC

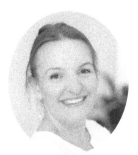

Ana discovered Chiropractic after leaving her studies in her 4th year at Medical School. In 2007 she graduated Summa Cum Laude at Life University where she fell in love with the Inside-Out paradigm. After graduation she opened her first practice and has been serving in her community in a high volume vitalistic practice since then. She is passionate about teaching students and other DCs through Technique, Philosophy and coaching. Known by her closest people as "tsunami", she focuses her energy in creating more ways to help people live the gift of the Inside-Out paradigm

What movies can teach us about Chiropractic

What a privilege and an honour to be part of this project. I hope this chapter brings a smile and some reflections for many.

Life feels like a movie sometimes and Chiropractic is about life, so let's take it from there and bring some movies into the picture.

I have to admit I am a Lord of the Rings fan and, like a good chiro freak, I see similarities everywhere. Gandalf would have been an amazing chiropractor. He understood life. Here are some of his most famous quotes:

"I will not say: do not weep; for not all tears are an evil".

What a great analogy for symptoms. Don't you think? I know he is not thinking about sciatica or migraines at the moment, but he is definitely talking about expressing all we feel, about not judging what is good or bad with our minds, or pretending to know what is supposed to be better or supposed to be happening. It takes courage to feel everything and to trust, no doubt, but understanding that symptoms might be part of the healing process is such a great start.

"All we have to decide is what to do with the time that is given to us".

Not sure if you have watched the movies, but just to create context, Gandalf says this after another character says: "I wish I wasn't going through this right now." Does that sound familiar? How many of us say that on a regular basis? And our clients? This might just be a movie character but he offers us a lot of wisdom and power; like Viktor Frankl told us, the only freedom that cannot be removed from us is the freedom to choose how to live the situation that we are living. Be it a symptom, a pandemic, a patient complaining, opening a practice or running it. Choice gives power. We have the power to make the best of every situation, one second, minute, hour and day at a time.

"There is some good in this world, and it's worth fighting for!"

Definitely. Sometimes we feel like we are fighting against something too big. People don't get it, big Pharma is too big, in Spain we are not even recognised as a healthcare profession; and then I remember the concept of "one spine at a time". The Big idea. The impact of that small adjustment in one person... multiplied by all our practices. Aren't we changing the world? I have no doubt we are. We are doing something good; we are creating something beautiful and it's definitely worth doing.

"Some believe that it is only Great Power that can hold evil in check. But that is not what I have found. I found it is the small things. Everyday deeds by ordinary folk that keeps the darkness at bay."

I love this one because it is true for us and our patients. First, a great reminder for us that what we do every day counts to make this world a better place. All our daily habits are making us a better version of ourselves. Not the once-a-year big thing, but mostly, the 5-minute things, done daily, of course. We are inspiring our clients every day to do the same thing. Regular adjustments, creating new habits; the small things, the everyday deeds. And maybe is not about fighting darkness but about keeping it at bay?

"It's a dangerous business going out your door. You step onto the road, and if you don't keep your feet, there's no knowing where you might be sent off to."

How many times a day do you push yourself out of your comfort zone? Growing is not easy. Part of our brain is designed to keep us were we are, comfortable. We wake every day, wanting to grow ourselves, our practices and to be better personally and professionally. But we also know "wanting" is not enough. Talking about it is not enough. We need to do something about it, one step at a time.

"It's the job that's never started that takes longest to finish."

This one makes me smile because again, this is so relevant for us and for our patients. We all want to grow, we all want to get better, but what about doing the work? We need to start and not all of us are willing to do that. I don't mean to judge anyone but it does take that first step.

That kind of stuff forces us to focus on the present and there is no better master than Master Oogway, in Kung Fu Panda, to teach us about the importance of the present.

"Yesterday is history, tomorrow is a mystery, but today is a gift. That's why it's called the present". I could quote this guy forever, but we are so good at staying present, one adjustment at a time, aren't we? We know the importance of being present with every single one of our clients. We have plans, goals, 10-year plans, but at the end of the day, we live in the present. We only have that; and what a gift.

In that present, we do the work. Sometimes not even seeing where it will take us. Frustrating at times, especially with long-term goals, not seeing immediate results. It takes so much work, doesn't it? Patients must be feeling the same way. Adjustment after adjustment. So what? Guess who felt the same way...

"Wax on, wax off".

If this doesn't sound familiar, I have no clue what age you are, but watch Karate Kid. It's about doing the work, every single day, trusting your teachers and mentors (and chiropractor?), and learning to think long-term without seeing the results right away. And yes, maybe one day we will understand why we were doing everything we were doing. This concept is big for our clients too. Helping them understand principle #6, what true health is and what we stand for in our profession is a little bit like, "wax on, wax off".

This profession is unique, because of our clear message: we cannot do it for you, but we can do it with you. Healing happens from the inside-out and we can remove the interference to the system in charge.

But not only that, we take the responsibility for that message and we understand that our growth also happens from the inside-out.

"With great power comes great responsibility".

Whether Uncle Ben in Spiderman is the first person to ever quote this is not relevant right now. Let's focus on the message. We are dealing with something powerful in our profession. An innate intelligence in every single organism and human being in charge of coordination, adaptation, healing and evolution. What a powerful concept. We understand people are in charge, we "just" remove that interference to the best of our abilities and the rest happens from the inside-out. That inside-out concept is what makes this profession so unique, to the point of making us look inside and be responsible for ourselves as well. We don´t take that responsibility for granted. We work on our ourselves, from the inside-out. We trust that there is something bigger, we grow, we are willing to do the work, starting with ourselves.

I don't know how many dentists, lawyers or surgeons go through the same type of mentorship and personal work we do. I really hope they do. We do because we work with that subtle thing and we understand what Uncle Ben, Spiderman's uncle, meant; it's not only "an adjustment", it's powerful, and we accept that responsibility.

And now, if I had to choose a quote to finish this article, I am definitely choosing a classic and something that makes me think of all of you, all these colleagues I have around the world. People I share principles with. People I love, because they love the same things I love.

"I think this is the beginning of a beautiful friendship". And project. For the millennials, this quote is from the movie Casablanca.

Wisdom #22

Greg Venning DC, CCWP

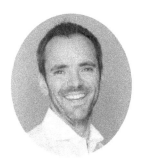

Greg is an author, wellness chiropractor, inspirational speaker and self-confessed "health geek". Following his own health challenges, he has dedicated his life to helping people fully express their human potential, working as a chiropractor and international speaker.

He is a certified Chiropractic Wellness Professional, an Advance Biostructural Correction Instructor and has completed a certification in Neurolinguistic Programming. Greg is founder of Peak Chiropractic Centre in Cape Town, South Africa and his motto is to help others to "live your bigger life". His first book, Thrive! is about creating a vitalistic lifestyle.

Experiencing "that moment"

It's been 30 years since my first chiropractic adjustment and as I think back over that time, I often wonder how different my life would be without it. You see, I really did fall into Chiropractic; I married a chiropractor. And while it was never my intention to work in Chiropractic, here I am 30 years later with 27 years' service, wearing many different chiropractic hats.

Chiropractic has given me more than just great health; it has given me the principles with which I choose to live my life. Without those principles, where would I be living? What work would I be doing? Would I have 6 children? What kind of medication would I be taking? The list goes on.

What I do know is that I have a certainty and belief in Chiropractic that guides me in everything I do. For me, living my life by chiropractic principles is just so simple and yet I live in a world watching others struggle with not only their health but their beliefs around health. I see a sense of powerlessness around life and an inability to make choices and decisions. I see people and communities not able to trust the innate wisdom of their bodies. Instead, they are fearful and often make health decisions from that place.

One question I often ask myself is, "Why doesn't everyone get it, how can they not see that life can be done differently?"

I have a distinct memory of the moment, yes that moment, the one when you "get it", when you really understand Chiropractic.

That moment when you know that we are self-healing, self-regulating organisms.

That moment when you know that your body has an inborn intelligence and we need to learn to tune-in to it.

That moment when you know that healing takes time.

That moment when you know that we are connected above down and inside out.

My moment wasn't via my mentor's teachings, nor his report of findings or even the fact that I had dramatic changes to my health. No, it was a moment in time when I was ready. I had spent time healing, learning, and most of all questioning everything I knew and understood about health.

There I was at a chiropractic conference and it hit me like a bolt of lightning. I had been listening to the same stories, the same information that I had heard many times before, but this time it was different. Chiropractic moved from being a treatment for ailments, to a way of life.

I am grateful for that moment. It has given me a life I could never have dreamed of. Not only have I had the great privilege of helping many people discover the benefits of Chiropractic in my varied roles, I have also had the great privilege of raising 6 beautiful chiropractic children. All born at home with no intervention, no vaccinations and only a handful of A&E visits. Being part of their journey to discovering their own views on health and the principles with which they "do life" has been and still is my greatest joy.

My wish for Chiropractic is that chiropractors gently lead their patients and communities to arrive at "that moment". That they don't just rely on that awesome pre-care class or report of findings. That they give them time and as Bill Esteb says, "Allow them the space to fail".

My wish for our future world is a life lived without fear, a life where we trust in the innate healing ability of the body. A life where people have tools to make decisions and choices aligned with their values and beliefs. Chiropractic has given me all of these things in abundance and I will always be truly grateful for "that moment".

Alison Young BChiro, BAppSci, MScAPP (Paeds)

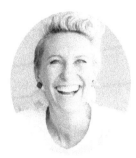

Dr Ali Young is a Chiropractor with a passion for serving children and families. She has completed a Masters in Chiropractic Paediatrics. Through her own motherhood journey, she has become passionate about connecting mothers with their inner vitality and their ability to regulate their environments purely with learning about themselves. She teaches online courses through her platform UnFck Motherhood and has an extremely busy private chiropractic practice in Gladstone Queensland Australia.

The principle of integration, motherhood and Chiropractic

"Reconnecting (wo)man the physical with (wo)man the spiritual"
– DD Palmer

The Motherhood journey is a complex rite of passage that women move through. Whether they become a biological parent, adopt, or are a step-parent, the transition into motherhood creates a large change in a woman's body; emotionally, physically and spiritually.

As chiropractors we are blessed to work with the intelligence that exists in the human body on a daily basis, witnessing miracles and supporting our people to express their lives fully. The core premise of innate intelligence, the intelligence that resides within us giving life and allowing us to function Above, Down, Inside, Out, really does give life form to our mothers. DD Palmer touched on it perfectly when he stated that as chiropractors, we are blessed to reunite man the physical with man the spiritual; and it is this concept that sets us apart!

The passage of a woman from womanhood to motherhood is a complex time, physically, emotionally and spiritually. The alteration in hormones is immense and has been likened to the changes that occur in a woman's body with adolescence, that huge shift that has been given so much time, research and regard. This hormonal and psychological shift of motherhood is labelled matrescence and is an evolving element of discovery for researchers worldwide.

As Chiropractors, we often work with mothers in the prenatal area; working at establishing a beautiful state of ease and connection, and balance within the system to really allow them to have the birth they want. A key element is supporting them in choice, to explore the ideas of birth, and to become aware of the power that lies within them, that allows them to be themself. The fundamental concept of, "You Do You".

And I feel that as a profession we do this so well. We provide a sense of confidence and trust within them that they may not get anywhere else. We outsource key literature, we recommend support workers such as midwives, doula's, hypnobirthing practitioners, naturopaths, Chinese medicine practitioners and herbalists, all with a key philosophy that the body works perfectly if it has no interference. In some places around the world, we are even a key component of the birthing team, helping in holding the space, supporting the mother and her partner and being there to be a guiding light. For this we are truly blessed.

However, and myself included in this, there is a space where our shift then moves to caring for the neonate. Caring for this wee babe that has entered this plane of the universe, and is so loved and wanted and cherished. And in this moment, we forget the mother. We forget to honour the journey that she has been through, the massive shift that has occurred within herself on a physical, emotional and spiritual level. And for us as chiropractors, the support of this shift, this is when her whole being has changed. This is our time to truly support a woman's integration into motherhood.

This is matrescence.

We are the answer to supporting this shift, as reuniting woman the physical with woman the spiritual, through our adjustment, our support and our understanding, is where true motherhood-focused care springs from. Not only before the birth, but the provision of love-focused care into this journey of motherhood and beyond.

The core premise of the big idea, that we are more than physical parts, but we are our intelligence, our interaction with the world, and our universal state, allows us to take a world view of this shift. The feeling of being in flow in practice, of that connection with the big "what is", this is where we can change some lives.

Mothers really need to feel understood. One of the greatest changes we are seeing in our world is the increase in postnatal depression and anxiety, with Australian women (AIHW 2012) reporting a 1 in 5 statistic in 2010, which has likely increased in recent times. In 2018 a retrospective study was conducted on Australian women (Ogbo etal), discovering that the risk factors for maternal depression were: lack of partner support, history of intimate partner violence, being from the Culturally and Linguistically Diverse population, and a low socioeconomic status. Postnatal depression was also being caused by assisted delivery, it found. Overall, the key elements affecting depression were demographic and psychosocial disadvantage.

If there is one space that we can work on as chiropractors, it is helping to promote a woman's worth within herself. Connectedness with self is where we can help them realise their true strength, and support them through this time. Removing physical pain, but more than that, allowing their body to be supported through the matrescence shift, this is our privilege.

So how do we do this? I'm not going to espouse one style of adjustment over another, one style of practice over another. We can be man or woman, solo or group practice, these factors don't define our success. What I am going to talk about is presence, energy and connectedness.

I remember going to my first Parker seminar in Melbourne, and Fabrizio was discussing PTC. I'd heard it before, I thought I owned it, but it's not until you experience really being there for that person, the only thing of your focus, that you get that presence. That connection of yourself to the big world and to them, all at the same time. That sense that you just "know" what is happening, the intuitive focus.

As a practitioner who started working just as mobile phones were becoming a thing, the evolution of the distraction we all experience has been significant. Conscious awareness of not being distracted is necessary in the age of tech that we are living in. It's subconscious for us to think about where the next image for our clinic social media platform is coming from, what story can we share, what engagement have we had with our latest practice or personal post; and has my partner called. We need to be consciously aware that when we are in service mode, that is exactly what we do.

Both our practice members, and ourselves need us to show up completely. Be 100% present for them when it is their time, and you will begin to see how the intuition of "knowing" floods back to you, and the care that those mothers need will begin to occur. The subtlety of a change when they are chatting with you about it all, the sense that they need a big cry, are to be truly listened to. This ability to tap in, it all comes from presence.

Energy is a fluid motion, back and forth. We've all felt it, that awkward space when walking into a room when a couple has just had a disagreement; going in to check a newborn baby when one parent doesn't want them assessed; or the partner who has been sent to your practice on their own, with no idea why. A mother's energy is often in 20 places at once, so holding that space of care and concern for her, enables her energy to being to categorise itself into a sense of order. Listening to her words and really being there for her will allow that energetic focus to occur.

This doesn't have to take long; you can become an energy ninja. Finding chiropractors to observe and sense this ninja status, that really uplevelled my game. You also need to learn how to be protective of your energy. Just like in the song the Gambler, *"You've got to know when to hold 'em, know when to fold 'em"*.

It's pretty much the same. You need to know when it's time to use yours to settle a space, and when you need to protect your own, in order to conserve and preserve your energy. One thing that's key for a chiropractor is to make sure they are adjusted, as when you're on a level playing field, you have that ability to control your energy at the right level.

Working with mothers, I find they're commonly energy depleted or running in sympathetically dominant "manic" mode. Being able to meet them where they're at, and slowly bring them up through the adjustment, through allowing the flow of them to the connection of the universe, this is our gift. Holding space, and using our adjustment and touch to support this system to energetically level, is prudent.

Connection with the mother comes from the space of deep awareness of what they are going through, of understanding that things are hard right now, and that you can help them journey through it. This is the core to working with mums and supporting them through the matrescence that they go through postnatally.

Yes, they may have a beautiful baby, but they may not necessarily feel endless love towards it. Societal pressure means there's an expectation that we will love our babes fiercely and unconditionally as soon as we birth them, and that anything less is a failure. But it doesn't always happen like this and that drives a lot of the up-and-down that women regularly report to me. The feeling of failure. They may not feel they are doing a great job, or even a good job. They may have a babe who is stamping their authority on their entry into the world, with more crying than rest. Mums have often invested plentiful hours planning their birth, and the space that the baby will be coming home too, but haven't really delved into the whole concept of loss and gain of their old life, of endless love but filled with frustration; the whole dichotomy that is mothering.

But if you, as a chiropractor, can help them feel connected with their own intuition, if you can clear interference and provide physical relief, offer support that allows them to trust their instincts, and possibly link them with other providers, then this is true motherhood care.

I love that I am in a profession that has a true philosophical construct, that the universal intelligence uniting with innate is really where expressing our life fully is at. To me, there is never a greater time to be part of the journey of a fellow human than in this sphere of motherhood. Thanks for taking this journey with me, and for providing the utmost amazing care for the matrescence of these amazing women.

Wisdom #23

Selina Sigafoose DC

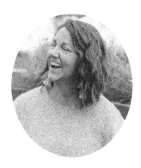

Having grown up in a family of chiropractors, Selina graduated from Life Chiropractic College in 1989. She met Kevin Jackson on the second day of school and they married in July 2, 1988. Together they run a large practice in York, Pennsylvania and share two stunning daughters, Kinna and Kloé, a son-in-law, Austin and a new grandson, Haddon James Shaffer.

Wanting to enjoy every aspect of her life, Selina's goal after sharing her 12-14 minute new patient orientation is to leave them saying "WOW". She is a founder of The League of Chiropractic Women and serves as the first female Vice President of the ICA.

My experience of Chiropractic

I, Selina Sigafoose Jackson, am blessed to have been raised by an amazing chiropractic philosopher, James M Sigafoose DC. Being raised by such a man has created within me the desire to see all of life through the lens of spirituality. So, in Chiropractic, all I know are the laws of life. That all things occur first in the spiritual realm, then manifest in the physical. Therefore, when I read and study the 33 principles, I see them through a spiritual lens. My lens. I have a few that are my favourite.

Principle #1: Major premise. A universal intelligence is in all matter and continually gives to it all its properties and actions thus maintaining it in existence. Wow! Is that not exciting? Can we doubt our existence? Can we doubt our journey? Can we doubt our success or our failures? Yes, we can doubt but if we believe one part of the principles, we must believe them all and thus Principle #1 states that the intelligence in us, our Creator, is in us, giving to us, maintaining us. That is so hopeful, encouraging, powerful, everlasting. We have all the tools necessary to achieve all we choose. It does require discipline. It does require an understanding that, depending on the journey, we are called to a different standard. A higher standard. A standard that requires one to seek, learn, be quiet and still to hear and be brave enough to act. Act in a way that brings honour to this intelligence and principle. That looks different for each of us but it is laced with respect, mercy and grace.

My next favourite is Principle #11: The character of universal forces. The forces of universal intelligence are manifest by physical laws. They are unswerving and unadapted and have no solicitude for the structures in which they work. This principle can be looked at in multiple ways. I look at it as, there is an intelligence within that is moving forward with or without us. The Creator has a plan and it is happening whether we agree or disagree, understand, care or plan. My thought is that if we get on board with the plan by quieting and surrendering to the voice within, innate, and allowing life to unfold as our Creator is moving us, then life will be so much more peaceful then fighting, being selfish, and making excuses for successes or failures. Not all things that occur are sunshine and roses but they occur regardless. There is absolutely a time to fight and a time to surrender. We will know and understand this with clarity if we seek to quiet ourselves and listen to the wee small voice that we all have within, if we are willing to humble ourselves and be disciplined to back away from the world and be still.

It is truly easier than we make it. It is harder to fight against universal intelligence. We are all created to desire a connection to something higher and bigger than ourselves. It is innately and genetically inbuilt in us. Many choose to drown it out by filling it with social media, news, TV or material goods. That requires far more work and striving than to just shut it all down and be still and quiet. Be patient and wait. Be sincere and gracious. Our Creator, universal intelligence, wants a relationship with us. We just have to slow down and be humble and quiet long enough to let the world pass by and earn a conversation with one who has given us all our properties and actions, thus maintaining us in existence. One who will not swerve or adapt and will fight for us to run this race of life and finish powerful, strong and courageous.

Which brings us to Principle #6: The principle of time. There is no process that does not require time. If we continue to seek, surrender, be still, quiet, listen and then act on what we have been given, the law of time will prove that we have done our due diligence. It will see and reap the rewards of all that we are willing to say no to, and all we are brave enough to say yes to.

These 33 principles are filled with more truth and direction than we know. I encourage us all to dissect and study them and create a life plan and action with them to create the life we deserve, as a child of the most awesome!

Kevin Jackson DC

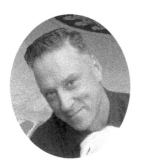

Canadian born Kevin graduated from Life University as a DC where he met and later married his wife Selina Sigafoose with whom he shares two daughters, Kinna and Kloé who are both studying to be chiropractors.

They currently own and operate one of the largest chiropractic practices in the United States and have done so for the past 30 years. Kevin is the Vice President of his state chiropractic organisation the Chiropractic Fellowship of Pennsylvania. He is also a Fellow of the ICA and is highly sought as a speaker at chiropractic events around the world.

What makes chiropractic unique

For me, Kevin Jackson, Chiropractic always has and hopefully always will be a separate, unique, and distinct healing profession dedicated to the analysis, detection and correction of the vertebral subluxation complex.

The vertebral subluxation complex is the only legitimate explanation for the condition that a patient seeks chiropractic care and the specific adjustment the only legitimate procedure that has allowed people to express greater potential. Whether that greater potential is through health, academics, athletics, or any other human endeavour.

Ask any practicing chiropractor if the overwhelming majority of their patients have had their simple or complex health conditions clear up and the answer is unequivocally "yes".

Ask any chiropractor who practices family care, if the

school age children and young adults who get maintenance adjustments miss less school, get better grades and seem to do better academically, and the answer is unequivocally "yes".

Ask any chiropractor who has ever taken care of athletes from the little leagues through professional levels, if these athletes get injured less and perform at their best. The answer is always the same; unequivocally "yes".

Chiropractic has survived and thrived throughout the last 125 years not from support and money from pharmaceutical companies, not from grants given by wealthy business tycoons or celebrities and not from huge endowments from being part of a massive public university system. Chiropractic has survived and thrived based on the public getting results from chiropractors practicing a separate, unique, and distinct principle.

The principle of Chiropractic is a basic fundamental truth in that the human body is a self-healing and self-maintaining organism. The self-healing and maintaining is almost exclusively carried out by 2 branches of the central nervous system, the sympathetic and parasympathetic systems.

A healthy body goes through the day monitoring its environment through the sensory part of the nervous system, signalling all possible needs to the brain. After the brain receives and processes the needs of the body, it sends the appropriate and proportionate functional directive through the motor nervous system. This sensory input and motor output makes up the basic neurological loop. This intact and uninterrupted neurological loop keeps the body in a state of homeostasis.

Back in 1895, a healer known as DD Palmer first identified a possible break in the neurological loop that can occur due to physical, mental, or chemical trauma. He named this interruption of the normal state of nervous system function as the vertebral subluxation complex (VSC). Basically, the VSC creates a weakness within the body and does not allow the body to adapt to its ever-changing environment.

It is this concept or philosophy that immediately became at odds with the practice of medicine at the time. Medicine stated that the cause of disease was from germs or conditions outside the body, while Chiropractic stated that dis-ease, sickness, and decreased potential was created inside the body. At its roots, medicine and chiropractic are didactically opposed.

In modern times it has been established that the truth is somewhere in between. While we need to have clean water, air, food supply and sanitation, we equally need to understand the complex neurophysiology of the human body and what we might do to keep structure and functional heath at its optimum.

This is where the separate, unique, and distinct principle and practice of Chiropractic becomes an indispensable procedure and lifestyle for the modern day needs of a heavily polluted planet. Since we cannot control the external environment that we live in, it's imperative and non-negotiable that we try to control and optimise our internal environment.

There is abundant current and available research to support the vertebral subluxation complex, with virtually no current research denying its existence. Chiropractic is not thought or taught to be the cause of disease. Chiropractic adjustments are not thought or taught to heal disease. Chiropractic is a separate, unique, and distinct service offered by chiropractors only to adjust the vertebral subluxation complex to allow optimal neurological expression. Chiropractors understand that the nervous system controls and coordinates all bodily functions.

Chiropractors believe everyone could benefit by being checked for the presence of the vertebral subluxation complex and receive a chiropractic adjustment only when indicated and necessary.

Tim Young DC

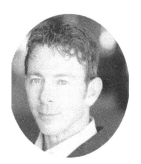

A proud father of 3, Tim was born and raised in Springfield, Missouri. After graduating in 1994 from Cleveland Chiropractic School in Kansas City, Tim and his family relocated to Oklahoma City where he began his own practice, Young Chiropractic.

Currently the Founder and past president of The Oklahoma Chiropractors' Association and Founder and President of the national chiropractic education seminar company Focus OKC, Tim travels around the world with his Chiropractic Mastery programme, teaching specific adjusting technique and patient connection.

What Chiropractic is to me

"Your chiropractic adjustment is your signature and defines who you are as a chiropractor." – Dr Hugo V. Gibson

Chiropractic is defined as a science, philosophy and an art. In today's Chiropractic, the science is pushed very hard, mainly because all you have to do is read and memorise, it's easier to teach. The philosophy is extremely diminished because it requires much contemplation, debate and thought. Who has time for that? But the art, the art of Chiropractic or the adjustment, is all but lost in the profession. The art of the adjustment is like no other. It takes a great deal of practice, focus and self-realisation to come to an understanding of just how profound the act of adjusting the human spine actually is.

I graduated from Cleveland Chiropractic School in 1993, back in the old days when they still referred to it as a Chiropractic school. I feel I was very fortunate, but also unknowingly witnessing the end of an era. As students, we had the privilege, like so many before us, to have professors such as Hugo Gibson and Muriel Perillat who actually had successful practices and understood chiropractic on a much deeper level. There was still an enormous stress being put on the 3 pillars of Chiropractic, at least by a few of the professors. The adjustment was just as important, if not more so than the science or philosophy.

We, as students, understood that if you could not deliver the adjustment you would always struggle in practice. My uncle graduated from Cleveland in 1966. He told me that back then, if you couldn't deliver a proper adjustment to the satisfaction of the clinicians at that time, you didn't graduate until you could. The attitude was that it was the school's responsibility to see to it that doctors going out into the public were well trained, effective and safe. If you have ever watched old videos of past chiropractic adjusting labs, you can quickly tell that it was a very intense and important part of the learning experience.

Today, the specific chiropractic adjustment has been reduced to a gross manipulation and taught to be feared as dangerous and not as essential as it once was. I have travelled the world for the past 10 years working with chiropractic students and field doctors on adjusting technique. I listen to their stories and observe their skill levels and I am always shocked to see what is being taught as an adjustment. It's sometimes overwhelming for me to witness the lack of skill and understanding, as well as the fear that has been instilled into these young doctors. This also explains the large number of failing practices, as well as the enormous emphasis on other therapies. I once read a statement from a practicing chiropractor that read, "*The chiropractic manipulation is just something that some chiropractors do sometimes along with other therapies.*"

When I was a first-year student, I had an experience that changed me forever. I was in Dr Gibson's full spine adjusting class. We called it the Meric technique back then. The technique required a very intense study of the spine, facet angles, set up, lines of drive etc. This technique might be called "toggle" today. Dr Gibson is what we called "old school" because he was and still is one of the most principled chiropractors I have ever met. By principled I mean he has a very deep and personal understanding of the 3 pillars of Chiropractic, not only as a professor but as a practicing chiropractor.

During the final exam, we all had to set up on a patient and deliver an adjustment. It had to be perfect in Dr Gibson's eyes or you did not move on from his class. I had been given the 5th lumbar on the right side. As I set up on my patient and prepared to make my adjustment, I looked up and saw Dr Gibson standing directly in front of me. His eyes where focused and intense. Just as I was about to deliver the adjustment, he said in his very deep South African accent, "Feel it in your soul lad." It was, in my mind, still the best adjustment I ever gave.

Feel it in your soul. Why was that statement so profound that it still echoes in my head all these years later? The chiropractic adjustment, when delivered appropriately, is an extension of the chiropractor's soul. A very intimate piece of who and what they are. It is not to be taken lightly or disregarded as a mere therapy. The chiropractic adjustment is a gift from God to mankind. The adjustment has the power to allow healing within anyone and anywhere. I have witnessed chiropractic offices where patients park in a parking garage and pay, walk down a steep hill, receive an adjustment and walk all the way back up the hill. I have witnessed the elderly walk 3 flights of stairs to a chiropractor's office to receive their precious adjustment.

In my own office I have witnessed people drive up to 5 hours one way, receive an adjustment that takes less than 30 seconds and then drive home, happily. I have witnessed a very sick and struggling newborn in a neonatal intensive care unit immediately come back to life after a very specific and intentional chiropractic adjustment.

The art of the adjustment should be mastered and revered as a unique gift. We as chiropractors have been blessed to share this gift with the world. I see thousands of chiropractors selling their finger-painting versions of an adjustment and attempting to pass them off as Rembrandts. I believe as a profession that until we shift our emphasis back to balancing the 3 pillars, science, philosophy and art, we will never reach our full potential as leaders in the healthcare arena.

Alasha Young DC

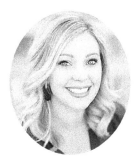

Alasha went to the University of Oklahoma where she studied Pre-Chiropractic and Health and Exercise Science. She received her Doctorate in Chiropractic from Parker University in 2017.

She is certified in Webster Prenatal Technique, is a Birthfit professional, EPIC Pediatric certified and an active member of ICPA.

All it takes is love

"I give with the only thing I have, love. And I love all by removing that which interferes with 100% life. I do not look to others for direction, I look within. I am a perfect expression of God living 24 hours each day for others – I am a principled Chiropractor." - BJ Palmer, DC, Ph.C

"I love all by removing that which interferes with 100% life."

These are the words that I say to myself many times a day. They ground me, they inspire me and they empower me. Chiropractic awakens and turns on life through the art of adjustment; it frees people and allows them to express health at their fullest potential. Chiropractic is such a beautiful thing and I'm filled with gratitude that it found me. It found me through my father and has guided me through my life. If I didn't have chiropractic, it would be hard for me to comprehend how drastically different my life would be. It's not what I do, it's who I am.

To be honest there was a time that I didn't want to be a chiropractor. Through my journey as an undergraduate I was searching for my own passion. I searched for something that fueled my soul, something that could change others' lives, something that could have a huge impact on the world. I wanted to find that something that created the joy which Chiropractic created in my father's heart and eyes. I searched, but I couldn't find it; Chiropractic had found me. It spoke to me, it called me and now I have a deep burning love for Chiropractic.

When I was an undergraduate and finally accepted the fact that I was meant to be a chiropractor, my heart jumped for joy. A couple weeks into chiropractic school I was distraught. "What is this, where am I? What do you mean we aren't allowed to adjust? We are going to fail? I'll get kicked out of school for adjusting? I have to use therapies to be successful? I should specialise in something, because chiropractic isn't enough? I should only treat one area? I shouldn't take X-rays? When is someone going to talk about adjusting moms and babies? It's 6 visits and refer out? I'm going to get sued? When are we going to talk about miracles?"

This Chiropractic that others were talking about wasn't the same Chiropractic I knew. I was heartbroken. This amazing thing that I knew deep inside me, that changed my life, may have been different to what I thought it was. Soon after, I was approached to go on a chiropractic mission trip to Cap-Haïtien. Was my technique ready? No. Was my heart crying out for me to go? Yes. My soul spoke to me and said, "You must go." When that happens, you should always listen.

When I got to Haiti, I was asked by one of the mentoring chiropractors, "What do you want?" I replied, "I want to be an amazing chiropractor, I want to serve children, because chiropractic changed my life as a child." That day I got to serve hundreds of children. People were lining up and fighting over the chiropractic adjustment. People were crying out about how the chiropractic adjustment had changed their life. That day, a 2-year-old little girl named Lovelie and her 7-year-old sister watched me adjust for hours.

Lovelie's older sister held her, as she couldn't walk. She was malnourished, covered in dirt, and the only clothes she had were swimsuit bottoms. The biggest thing I noticed about Lovelie was that she was unable to make any connection with her eyes. The older sister tried to bring Lovelie to me multiple times, but she was not accepting. After everyone left that day, the older sister tried one more time. The older sister laid Lovelie on my table. Lovelie was calm as I palpated her upper neck and felt a lateral right atlas. As a young student I had never been more sure about a subluxation. It was almost as if I could feel it through my whole body, it actually scared me. I slowly reached down and adjusted Lovelie while looking into her eyes. Lovelie immediately looked back into my eyes. It was as if I could feel the pulse of the earth beneath my fingertips. A voice within me said, "Give with the only thing you have, love. And love all, by removing that which interferes with 100% life." From that day on I have never questioned the power of true chiropractic.

Wisdom #24

Skip and Judy Wyss DC, Caccp

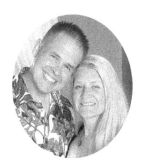 *Dr Skip Wyss and his lovely wife, Dr Julie Wyss reside in Green Bay, Wisconsin. They have an amazing pediatric practice that sees 70% children. Their office specialises in women of all ages and very young men. They both have certifications in pediatrics and pregnancy, and also the Webster's Technique through the International Chiropractic Pediatric Association. They are 2008 graduates of Palmer College of Chiropractic. Dr Skip is the co-creator of the PRIME Pediatric Program and creator/host of the PRIME Pediatric Podcast. He is a teacher and coach for the Practice Evolution Program where creating extraordinary family chiropractors is paramount. He is an internationally recognised speaker and author in the pediatric chiropractic realm.*

Dr Julie is Executive Director and co-founder of the non-profit organisation The Spine Project with her husband. She is a regional director for BIRTHFIT and the powerhouse behind the brand The Momma Phoenix which supports women, particularly during the postpartum transition to helping them feel connected and authentic.

We offer hope...

When asked for words of wisdom, our thoughts immediately go back to graduate school; we received no words of wisdom. We received many thoughtful words of encouragement and were told to plan for a long and arduous beginning, that hopefully we could weather the storm and tough it out. We were told all the stats on how many small businesses close or go bankrupt within their first year. But let's back up for a moment.

Hi, I'm Julie and I'm Skip! We are a husband-and-wife team who are both certified and sought-after pediatric chiropractors. We actually didn't meet in graduate school, we met as undergraduates in a microbiology class of all places. We both knew that we wanted to be chiropractors and were pretty certain that we didn't want to work for anyone else. Fast forward 2 years and we were in our last trimester of graduate school. We were newly married and excited about finishing school. One month later we found out we were expecting! To say that everything was turned upside down would be a good description. Little did we know that things happened just as they were supposed to.

After graduating, we moved back to our home state of Wisconsin and to an entirely new city. We had no connections, no family, no resources. We had each other and a precious new baby girl who we had to provide for. We managed to get a bank financed loan after being turned down by at least 12 banks; we were opening our office in the 2008 recession after all.

Now, back to those words of wisdom. We had no words of wisdom given to us. Everyone, our teachers, doctors, staff, family, they all offered us doubt, talked about hardships and sacrifice. No one talked about hope and success. It was not until we hit the lowest of lows in our first 4 months in practice that we realised that those doubts and words were what was holding us back. As soon as we dropped that baggage and made the conscious choice to surround ourselves with those of success, intention and character, we were able to flourish. And flourish we did!

We have the top pediatric office in our state, hold distinguished certifications and are a beacon to the families in our community. Year after year we continue to gain momentum in our community and are a million-dollar pediatric and pregnancy practice. But we did not become successful the way people might think. We do not market. We do not sell. We offer hope. Our patients are the key to our success; well, that and our expertise, knowledge, and skills!

Let us touch on that for a moment. What sets our office apart from most? Intention, passion, hope and results. Within these 4 processes, families' lives are changed forever, changing the trajectory of their childrens' lives as well as those of their future children, their future children's children and so on. That is how.

Intention: Doctors speak of the intention within an adjustment and how powerful it can be. When actively listening to a patient or seeing the pain deep within someone's soul and responding with a touch, a nod, or a reassurance, this is responding with intent. The intention to help and do no further harm. When anything is done with the right intent, you are living a congruent life.

Passion: Do you wake up every day loving what you get to do? Look forward to serving your patients on a higher level of healing? This is living your soul purpose. This is your life's passion. Living your life's passion should bring fulfilment and joy. It is different for everyone; family, money, travel. But if that passion is gone, then what good, what fun, is life? It is okay for your vision to change, it often does. Just be sure that whatever your next path is, it is congruent, served with intent and brings you passion.

Hope: Our world is on a search for hope. We're often told,

"you are our last resort, our only hope". Society as a whole has been maintaining, not thriving; just getting by. If you give just one person a glimmer of hope, that can turn into a cascading ripple effect. That person echoes the hope you have given them, which changes their energy and vibration. That next person feels it, has hope for that person as well and the cycle continues. But we cannot give hope without the ability to deliver. That comes from your skill set, knowledge, coaches, systems, and procedures. Your results should speak for themselves.

Results: This is one of those things that many people struggle with. Within Chiropractic so many have been misguided or lost. They have either never seen or learned about the amazing healing power of the body, or it is seen as no big deal. This is the division in our profession. Those who have not, and those who have, seen lives changed.

Scoliosis gone.

Hearing restored.

Seizures halted.

Arthritis reabsorbed.

Discs regenerated.

If one has never seen or experienced these things, it is no wonder they do not or cannot deliver the results their patients are looking for. You have given hope; now you need to deliver the goods!

Our office is sought out because of the results we get, but we deliver those results with intent, passion, and the vision of hope. The hope we give is built on a foundation of principles. As long as your intent and purpose are aligned, you will outlast any competition, natural disaster or devastation. The doctors that we teach and train will come and go but their foundation will remain, and they will live their life's passion and continue to deliver hope to their deserving communities.

A strong foundation will lead you to your life's passion. As long as you never falter, and deliver with love and intent, you will sleep peacefully at night. That is living in congruence with your mission and plan as God has intended. That is the Kids First brand!

We now make it part of our life's intent which has now, in turn, became our passion, to continue to spread the message of Chiropractic; but not solely to the greater masses as you might assume. The message needs to be brought to our brothers and sisters, our colleagues, and students.

Just like an adjustment given with the right intent, mentoring a student or new doctor with that same intent will begin to change the future of Chiropractic. Right now, it is seen as a dying art. Schools are dropping philosophy, removing the word Subluxation, pushing for Pharma rights. One of the latest recordings from the Prime Pediatric Podcast raised the question, "Are you willing to go to jail?" We ask you to truly consider this. If you are living within your sole purpose, full of passion for what you do, then you should be on fire, telling the world about the amazing healing potential of the body. Giving hope! Can you live without your life's passion? Could you live with the disappearance of Chiropractic? It is our duty to teach those who have never experienced the true power of Chiropractic. Be a mentor. It blows our minds how much we had to do to get ahead. No one was willing to lend a hand. Any piece of advice came at a cost. Everyone considered you the competition; like there aren't enough patients to go around! Nothing could be further from the truth.

When you see your colleagues faltering, you need to step up and support. What ever happened to helping your brothers. It does no good to let one falter. It only affects the chiropractic profession. This is where our passion lies, in spreading the message of Chiropractic. To give hope and the tools to succeed, so that our doctors can continue to give hope to their communities and ultimately change the health of the world.

We are so humbly honoured to be able to do what we do, every day. We are living our life's passion. And so, should YOU!

Judy Campanale DC, ACP

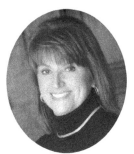

Past president of the IFCO, history-maker Judy owns and practices at the Strauss Chiropractic Center, in Levittown, Pennsylvania which is widely recognised as one of the longest-standing, high-volume, cash practices in the world (it celebrated 50 years in 2017).

Her contributions to Chiropractic are many and varied, including serving as editor of many of the Blue Books, written by Dr Joe Strauss. Since 2016, she has written the monthly ICPA Kids' Newsletter, Your Amazing Body, and served on the Board of Trustees of Sherman College of Chiropractic. She is currently Chair of the Board.

Shifting the focus

Early in my life, it was decided that I would be a doctor. It's true, I did well in school. I knew my colours in kindergarten, memorised the multiplication tables with ease in 2nd grade, loved science by 4th grade, and graduated at the top of my 8th grade class. I went on to study pre-med at Carnegie-Mellon University. I took the Medical College Admissions Test in my junior year and shortly after, developed significant abdominal pain. It would turn out to be significant in more ways than one.

To get to the bottom of the health challenge I was experiencing required 4 different doctors and 2 interns, on 3 separate occasions, at 4 different clinics and hospitals, with 2 grossly incorrect diagnoses. All of this led to a delay in my care and resulted in major surgery that would leave me unable to have children of my own later in life.

I share this personal information about me not to be dramatic, but to help you understand how I got to where I am in Chiropractic. Wisdom has been defined as *"the quality of having experience, knowledge, and good judgment; the quality of being wise."* I surely have that in this regard. It can also be defined as the body of knowledge and principles that develops within a specified society or period, and we are going to talk a little bit about that here.

From the very beginning, Chiropractic was developed as something different to medicine. Since the objective of medicine is the identification and treatment of symptoms and disease, that means that Chiropractic was intended to be something different to the identification and treatment of symptoms and disease. And it was. The founders of Chiropractic, in their wisdom, developed a set of principles that helped define and direct the practice of the early practitioners and the course of the future of the profession.

This is not to say that medicine is bad. There is surely a time and place for medicine, but its weaknesses are well known and well documented. It turns out that the weakness that changed the course of my life, misdiagnosis, was not so uncommon after all. As recently as 2014, the Mayo Clinic, undeniably one of the best in the business, still estimates their misdiagnosis rate at nearly 30%. Not knowing what the disease is presents a huge problem when your objective is the treatment of disease. Still, medicine's weaknesses will never make Chiropractic, or any other profession, good, right, or better.

Chiropractic, being different to medicine, has an objective that is different to medicine's. Chiropractic's objective is dictated by its founding principles, and follows both naturally and logically from the perspective that living things are self-healing. Living things express the principle of active organisation. Hence, Chiropractic looks at what is right with the body, not what is wrong with the body.

The principle of active organisation varies somewhat, but is deduced logically, from Chiropractic's major premise that all things, living and non-living, have an intelligence that determines their characteristics and maintains them in existence. The organisation itself suggests the intelligence.

Fortunately (or unfortunately), Chiropractic's principles have long been relegated to the philosophy arena. However, in a new and provocative book, A New Look at Chiropractic's Basic Science, Claude Lessard DC suggests that chiropractic's 33 principles are really the basic building blocks upon which we build our objective. Consequently, they determine and dictate (or should anyhow) our day-to-day practice. Lessard suggests that the 33 principles are really our basic science.

Truly there is a principle of organisation that is at work in each of us and in our world. The principle of organisation is as real and applicable as the principle of gravity. No one suggests that gravity is a philosophy; it is considered science. Whether you can prove it or not, or believe it or not, the principle of gravity is at work. You might be thinking, "Well yeah but we've done a lot of research on gravity!" That is true, but understand that the principle of gravity was the same before that fateful day when Sir Isaac Newton noticed an apple fall to the ground, as it is today. Gravity is and was a principle.

And just as gravity works on everyone and everything on earth, constantly attracting things downward to the planet, the principle of organisation too applies to everyone and everything. And just as the principle of gravity works whether you know about it, have studied it extensively, or don't even believe in it, so too with the principle of organisation. It does its thing whether you recognise it or not.

In living things, the principle of active organisation takes two little cells and grows them into an incredibly amazing little creature; in the case of people, a baby. It may seem like magic, but it is the result of a principle in action. More importantly, that principle of organisation doesn't stop expressing itself after birth. It continues to organise and maintain the living thing through all phases of growth and in every stage of life. This is what the chiropractor addresses and works with.

Chiropractic's Principle 20 states that a "living thing" has an inborn intelligence within its body, called Innate Intelligence. That is to say that every living thing exhibits the principle of active organisation. The purpose of that intelligence is to maintain the material of the body of a living thing in active organisation (Principle 21). More importantly, the principle of organisation is always expressed in the perfect amount. Just as the principle of gravity doesn't sometimes leave the apple floating in air or falling so hard that it crushes through the earth, the principle of active organisation is expressed in the requisite amount, proportional to its organisation (Principle 22).

Of course, all living things are constantly subject to a multitude of various forces which can be destructive to them. The function of the principle of active organisation is to adapt universal forces and matter for use in the body, so that all parts of the body will have co-ordinated action for mutual benefit (Principle 23). It does this in living things as long as it can do so without breaking a universal law. This is the disclaimer that states that the principle of active organisation is NOT magic (Principle 24).

Other important characteristics of the principle include that the means by which the principle maintains active organisation are always in the living thing's best interest and never injure or destroy the structures in which they work (Principle 25). And that the expression of the principle of organisation is always normal and its function is always normal (Principle 27). These important principles are what give Chiropractic certainty. This is in stark contrast to the treatment of disease, which can and does do harm, certainly from misdiagnosis but also sometimes from appropriate treatment of the correct diagnosis.

Herein is the beauty of the separate and distinct objective of the chiropractic profession. The forces of the principle of active organisation operate through or over the nerve system in animal bodies (Principle 28). However, there can be interference with the transmission of innate forces (Principle 29).

Understanding that the principle of active organisation maintains the living thing in organisation in a perfect fashion, any interference to the principle would result in incoordination or dis-ease (Principle 30). This state could be described as lack of ease or less than ideal. Here is a part that some stumble on in Chiropractic's basics. Principle 31 states that interference with transmission in the body is always directly or indirectly due to subluxations in the spinal column. You may not buy that statement and it is true that there is no way to deduce or infer this statement from the previous, as many of the principles are. However, the fact remains, that any disruption would result in incoordination or less than ideal. Couple that with the fact that structure and function have an inseparable relationship, and it can be deduced that any change to the structure of the spine results in an undesirable effect of the nerve system.

And this is where the chiropractic principles stop. They do not present ideas about health. They do not suggest how to apply them as healing modalities. They do not present as an alternative to medicine. They simply state that a living organism can lack ease, coordination, or harmonious action of all the parts of an organism, in fulfilling their offices and purposes (Principle 32) in the presence of vertebral subluxation.

This is not to say that Chiropractic cannot be used to pursue a different objective. Plenty of modalities are used to accomplish various objectives. Some people use diet as a treatment for disease (ie diabetes, heart disease, cancer). Some use diet to obtain a particular outcome, for example building muscle for an athletic event. Others use diet because they know when they eat well, they sleep better, think better, and yes, feel better. In all of these cases, the diet may be the same, but the objective is different.

Make no mistake, your objective matters. Ask yourself, if a profession adopts an objective held by another profession, why would both be necessary? Chiropractic has a unique objective that makes it separate and distinct. This idea alone is what makes Chiropractic vitally necessary and may be the only thing that will ultimately ensure the future of the chiropractic profession.

To bring it all full circle, when I was misdiagnosed at the tender age of 19, I vowed that I would never do that to someone else. The beauty of chiropractic is that you need not dally in the precarious world of diagnosis. The job of the chiropractor is to identify and remove vertebral subluxation for a fuller expression of the principle of active organisation at work in all living things. The presence of vertebral subluxation is, in and of itself, a sole rationale for care and its removal undeniably increases the adaptability of living things in a positive way.

Chiropractors would thrive if they would educate people on how amazing their bodies actually are, that is, if they would stay focused on what is right with people's bodies. People, in general, focus on the one thing that isn't functioning properly or the way they would like it to, and lose sight of the miracle that is life.

Chiropractors could change lives if they would help people understand that living things are maintained in such an incredibly sophisticated and miraculous state of existence by a principle, the principle of active organisation.

What's more, the expression of that principle is inhibited by the presence of vertebral subluxation. This alone would have a significant life-changing effect and ultimately world-changing contribution to the planet.

Wisdom #25

Kevin Proudman DC, DO

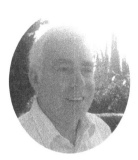

Kevin Proudman DC DO is a 1981 graduate of AECC who practices in Northern Ireland. He has opened and run 11 successful practices of which he has retained 2, where he employs and mentors associates. He served on the board of the British Chiropractic Association for several years, was a founding member of the United Chiropractic Association in 2000 and its second President, before serving on the General Chiropractic Council in the UK for five years after which he returned to service in the UCA, serving once gain as President for 11 years. He was voted Chiropractor of the Year in 2009 and oversaw the UCA's growth from a 'handful' of members to over 800. Dr Kevin is committed to keeping balance within the profession with a strong and deep-rooted conviction in vitalistic principles, administered through the medium of the spine and nervous system. He is a committed member of the Baha'i community for 45 years.

My 40 Years in Chiropractic

I feel honoured to have been asked to share some wisdom related to Chiropractic broadly centred on the 33 principles from RW Stevenson's book. These 33 principles helped form the foundation of the United Chiropractic Association when a small group of us brought it into being at the turn of the century. Despite the fact that I am in my 69th year and have been almost

40 years in full-time Chiropractic practice, I am a little bit wary to be claiming very much wisdom. I still feel I'm at the beginning of my education, the more I know the more I know I don't know, if you know what I mean.

I was born in England in the "Potteries" in 1951. I was an only child until I was 5 years old and we lived in the countryside, full of woods, rolling hills and steam trains. I enjoyed a good solid childhood with plenty of time on my own, especially enjoying reading and exploring. At the age of 10, I emigrated to Australia, with my parents and two younger brothers. We travelled on the Orion, a P&O cruise ship which had been used as a troop carrier during the Second World War and I still remember the 6-week journey with absolute joy. It was a fantastic adventure. We lived, initially, in the bush north-west of Sydney. Growing up in Australia was a great bounty. When I left school, I had a promising career in the bank of New South Wales, which lasted about 10 days. It was clear that my pathway was not office work or banking.

I then went to work at Channel 7 television in Sydney for a year. I did many other jobs in the short term, including working in a mining camp in the Gulf of Carpentaria and studying nursing. When I was 24 years old, I decided to become a primary school teacher. While studying at Goulburn teaching college, the most important thing to happen in my entire life occurred, which changed me immeasurably for the better. I was introduced to the teachings of Baha'u'llah by an old family friend. An almost physical and chemical change occurred in me as I embraced The Baha'i Faith with its teaching of the oneness of humanity and our responsibility in this life to be of service. To this day I am so grateful and I strongly recommend that you investigate it for yourself.

At the same time, I was introduced to some Baha'is who were also chiropractors. They suggested that I should look into Chiropractic as a career. Ralph Peters, Mary Ann Chance and Stanley Bolton, established chiropractors in Australia, all encouraged me. They took me to a public meeting in Canberra where 2 chiropractors from the United States, Buddy Grove and Lee Arnold, were doing a world tour lecturing on Chiropractic. After I listened to them there was no doubt that this was the pathway for my life.

Since I couldn't afford to go to the United States to study, and at the time there were no schools in Australia, I decided to go to Bournemouth in England to the Anglo European College of Chiropractic (AECC, at that time the only chiropractic school outside North America). I travelled to the UK in 1975 and started my studies in 1977. When I went for my first interview in Bournemouth, I met my classmate to be, Graham Heal who became my best and lifelong friend until his unfortunate death in a motorcycle accident. Graham's father had had an accident which left him quadriplegic. Attending a chiropractor, he first regained his sense of smell and then the use of his right arm. He was enabled to take up archery, winning a gold medal in the paraplegic games. He was also able to drive a car. His father's miraculous results were what led Graham to take up Chiropractic. For myself, I had never even had a Chiropractic adjustment before I entered college.

The education we received at AECC was of a very high standard as far as anatomy, neuroanatomy, histology, embryology and pathology were concerned. The word "subluxation" was never uttered.

There were two events which happened when I was at

AECC that helped me a lot. One was a visit by members of the Royal Commission from New Zealand who were investigating whether to accept chiropractic care into their national health service. The report they produced was excellent and very reinforcing as to the importance and efficacy of the profession and the importance and high standard of chiropractic X-rays. Well worth reading, and the result was that they did accept Chiropractic into their healthcare system. A member of their legal team was a lawyer, David Chapman Smith who was later to found the World Federation of Chiropractic (WFC).

The second event was a visit in our fourth year by Lee Arnold and Buddy Grove, again travelling the globe to promote the profession of Chiropractic. They were able to impart an understanding of chiropractic philosophy and vitalism to us which was clearly supported by scientific scholarship and professionalism. These two really served to generate enthusiasm about the possibilities of Chiropractic, although the ethos of AECC itself was (and still is) very medical and mechanistic. The class I started with had 52 students on the first day but by the end of the course we were reduced to about 23 graduates. Of my classmates, I think with the exception of 4 or 5 of us the majority did not really get the big idea of Chiropractic. For myself, I was lucky in that for the first year after graduation I worked with a Palmer graduate Dr Barry King, in Barnstaple in North Devon.

About 5 years after I graduated and following Barry's advice, I went to New York to a Parker seminar attended by 5,000 chiropractors. This gathering reinforced my enthusiasm for my profession which had been waning, crushed under the British chiropractic community's apparent need to be validated by the medical profession and its rejection of the traditions of Chiropractic. This negative attitude had already caused the split among UK Chiropractors, resulting in the formation of the Scottish Chiropractic Association and would later result in the foundation of the United Chiropractic Association. In New York there were 5,000 chiropractors gathered under one roof, all of them believing and confident in the efficacy of Chiropractic. It was very uplifting and reinforcing. At that time there were probably fewer than 1,000 chiropractors in the whole of Europe. When I returned to the UK after this conference, I resolved to try to expose my fellow chiropractors to the excitement and enthusiasm I had felt in New York. I did my best, but there was a well-organised political mission within a group of BCA grandees to medicalise the profession in the UK. This motivated small group has unfortunately managed over the ensuing years, to seize the levers of academic and regulatory authority within the profession in the UK.

Well, that's enough about me! What about some wisdom? I surely must have learned much in the last 40 years, having helped hundreds of thousands of patients regain and enhance their health through chiropractic adjustments. Having opened and established more than a dozen successful clinics, I have mentored and employed almost 100 chiropractors. I have also of course been a witness of history during this time.

Firstly, let's be very clear: Chiropractic is absolutely separate and distinct from modern medicine. In its essence, Chiropractic is within the vitalistic family of healing. That is to say it recognises and acknowledges the innate power and wisdom of the body to heal itself. The chiropractor's mission is to help with the expression of that innate power. In recognising that force, it is impossible not to also acknowledge that the individual innate intelligence is part of a universal intelligence which animates all living things. The healing that a chiropractor facilitates flows through him or her rather than coming from him or her. The chiropractor is a channel in that sense, nevertheless our education, skills and knowledge need to be of the highest quality to support that process.

I have seen healing miracles within my practice, as I know have many others. Great chiropractors in our history, people like Clay Thompson who invented the Thompson technique, Jim Parker who provided education through the seminars and who brought into being the Parker College of Chiropractic in Texas and many others, came to Chiropractic through these miracles. Clay Thompson for example was an engineer and in his middle years was diagnosed with a terminal illness. In desperation his wife sent him to a chiropractor and his results were so startling that he decided he must study and become a chiropractor. Jim Parker, as a 13-year-old had suffered conjunctivitis for many years, went to a chiropractor and after one adjustment woke the next morning thinking that he had gone blind, his eyes were completely glued shut with exudate. He washed his face and never again suffered from conjunctivitis.

These stories are multiplied by hundreds of thousands over the years and all over the world. The benefits of Chiropractic are nothing to do with the relief of pain in the back, neck and shoulder. The benefits of Chiropractic relate to the achievement of full potential by the individual, optimum health and the proper functioning of all the systems in the body. Chiropractors are nerve doctors, not bone doctors. As the chiropractor is working with the nervous system, the master control system, therefore the immune system, the endocrine system, the digestive system and all the other systems are helped to function more closely to their full potential.

In my experience chiropractors should have access to X-ray facilities. There is so much information which is useful to the patient in being able to visualise the structures with which you intend to work. The benefits far outweigh any very small risks. Unfortunately, there seems to have grown up a misunderstanding within the chiropractic profession regarding the necessity for imaging in the normal clinical setting. In my understanding, if at all possible, a chiropractor should strive to have X-ray facilities on site and to make the provision of quality radiographs a mark of excellence and pride.

Although there are many techniques and procedures which a chiropractor might use, they should always be congruent with your underlying principles. These principles or values are things like trustworthiness, honesty, kindliness, truthfulness, modesty, humility and service. Walt Disney is reputed to have said, *"When values are clear, decisions are easy."*

Always tell the truth (not least to yourself).

Other points which I hope you would find useful: avoid anger, stay out of consumer debt, investigate truth for yourself don't just believe others, always be willing to apologise, refrain from belittling others, try to go to bed at the same time as your spouse or partner at least 4 times a week, set worthy goals and serve others. I am sure (or I hope) I will have much more wisdom to share when I get old, but for now this will have to do.

An important event for the chiropractic profession in these islands will be coming to fruition quite soon: the establishment of a principled school of Chiropractic in Edinburgh. I hope everyone who wants to see a vibrant future for Chiropractic in the UK and Europe will put their wholehearted support into making the Scotland Chiropractic College a reality.

"DD Palmer - THE PERSON is not here now, He has come and gone but he left behind A PRINCIPLE, Chiropractic. As long as HE lived, HE protected his PRINCIPLE. Now that he - THE PERSON - is no longer here, it is OUR responsibility to protect, defend and preserve his PRINCIPLE. Once any PRINCIPLE becomes established, adopted and has become a part of and a necessity in daily life; like the car, electricity, aeroplane, it automatically lives in and from the inherent merit it possesses. Someday CHIROPRACTIC will do the same.

It is not so much a question of sincerity as it is WHO is MOST HONEST in sincerity and who is using BEST JUDGMENT with that sincerity. All leaders of men have been those who, in THEIR DAY, were RIGHT but HATED because THEY WERE RIGHT. Also, many men who were most LOVED have been pussy-footers, molly-coddlers, back-slappers, hand-shakers, who went about spreading platitudes to appease the egos of MOST men. We care not so much whether WE ARE LOVED so much as we are concerned in BEING RIGHT even THOUGH HATED because WE'RE RIGHT.

We should be kind, gentle, considerate and thoughtful of the rights OF PERSONS. We must be firm and just also in the defence of rights OF PRINCIPLES. The PRINCIPLE that can and does get sick people well IS CHIROPRACTIC

PERSONS who have THAT PRINCIPLE in their heads and hands MUST defend, protect and preserve THAT PRINCIPLE to preserve in it its purity for posterity to protect PERSONS' rights to application OF THAT PRINCIPLE so people CAN continue to get well after CERTAIN PERSONS pass on." *BJ Palmer*

Tiffany Johnson DC

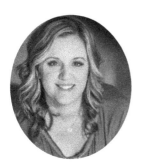 *Tiffany is a powerhouse chiropractor, podcaster, blogger and professional speaker. Based in West Fargo, USA, she spends her time raising her family and running a thriving chiropractic practice.*

Tiffany's passion lies in empowering other women through "The Aligned Life". This is her online business of memberships, courses, speaking engagements, group and one-on-one coaching focused on mindset, transformation and impact in all areas of life.

Getting the right team

Living and practicing in a way that is aligned to your soul's purpose may seem unattainable, but it's not. The truth is, there is no Aha-I've-made-it moment. Instead, you develop an alignment compass that tells you when you're moving towards alignment or away from it. The more we hide from ourselves and the quiet nudges, the further away from true alignment we are. Darkness needs to be brought into the light so it can heal; so it can be aligned and so that you can reach a point where you are truly living and loving in all areas of your life.

Your business is an extension of you. Your leadership style is an extension of you. Healing others is an extension of you. Running a successful business is about leading, communicating and selling. Of course, chiropractic technique is important, but it's not what will build trust, rapport and certainty. I'm going to share concepts and tactics about how to do this and how to make it scalable so that you aren't doing everything yourself.

Business alignment takes time, it's a journey and just as I mentioned above, there is no "I made it" moment but there is a steady progression towards it with every conversation, task and vision.

Here are my top 6 ways to build a sustainable high-volume and high-retention practice (and keep it for 15 years).

Confidence: You cannot focus on your team, patients, family, friends if you don't feel good enough in your skin. Evaluate your posture, how you walk into a room. You can't "fake it 'til you make it" in the confidence department. Know your gifts, know your challenges. Communicate and be vulnerable and stop being an actor. Be you, it's your journey to explore.

Chiropractic team: You need a chiropractic team. A support team. A personal team. If you want an office (and a life) that can be scaled, you need a team. Your team is the most important thing you can invest in. The gains that come from an efficient, trustworthy team will make up most of your expenses. There have been instances I've paid my staff before myself, knowing the only way I can get there is with them. The first to hire? Your concierge, your first-impression rose gal, the front desk chiropractic assistant (CA). The amazing human who answers the phone, greets everyone by name, runs all payments and handles back-end paperwork. That sounds so easy peasy! It's not necessarily easy, but is the first hire you need to make.

Here's a few tips on hiring:
- ✓ Hire for personality and train for skill.
- ✓ Always be on the lookout for prospects. The person who carries posture well, makes eye contact, has a rock star smile, has a grounded and loyal feel.

✓ Hire slow, fire fast and never avoid that gut feeling that something is off. Have the conversation right away so you don't deplete energy thinking and stressing about it.

Support Team: Banker, accounting, bookkeeper, attorney, cleaning, insurance agent. These people are part of your expert panel and you will gradually build this team.

Personal Team: Your spouse, family, kids, close friends because without them, life just isn't as awesome. You can be aligned in ALL areas of your life, but there will definitely be transitions; times where you will work more and others where you will play more. Be clear and communicate with the most important people in your life.

Systemise and train: No office is too small to create systems for every part of the business. Everything needs to be written down, saved and evaluated every quarter. We create these manuals in Google Docs so once they're saved and shared, any member can update it and it's saved on all devices. Here are some examples of the manuals we have:

Office Manual AKA Rules. With every new hire, they are required to read and sign off.

Front desk manual. This can be broken down further into open/close, new patient call, ROF prep, setting up payment schedule, etc.

Marketing manual
Social media manual
Billing manual
Bookkeeping manual

Delegate: Let go, my friend! Whether you're just starting your practice or scaling, delegation continues to evolve. This is one of the most difficult; letting go of control. Be clear in your expectations, train your staff appropriately and allow them to grow, expand and help you more. Help them live the life of their dreams while helping you reach yours. In order to create something unified, consistent and with expected results, it's imperative that you do what only you can do: adjust (well, there are maybe a few other things but you get the gist!). Know what your genius is and hire for everything else.

This exercise helped me: write a list of all the things that only you can do, then follow that with what you love to do. Some also like to add on what brings you profit. Find those few roles that are repeated. Those are your genius. This may be something you can implement immediately or it might be in your future plans. Whatever it is, consistently work towards that, communicate to your team so they know the vision and can help you get there. *Managing Up* by Jack Welch is a great book that breaks these concepts down well, for you and your team. I've been through this exercise a few times until I'm now only doing 2-3 things a day in my practice and everyone else is managing up. You can do this exercise with other docs, your office manager and any other roles. The goal is to have every person on the team working in their genius the majority of the time.

Build Rapport: It is your responsibility to know your people and their WHYs. They aren't in your office for Chiropractic per se, they're there because they are ready for change. Talk with them, not at them. Ask questions about their life, not just their pain. Give them hope and allow them to see possibility in their life. Learning who they are and what they really want will help them see that you may be the person to help them reach their goals. Know what matters to them, their goals, values and dreams; and meet them there.

Heart: Adjust with heart. Communicate with heart. Lead with heart. Listen with heart. Whether male or female, business owner or employee, a balanced approach is crucial. The masculine brain is logical, analytical, managerial. It's focused on decision making, financial considerations, goals, action, strategy, bottom line and running the team. The feminine brain is heart-centred, intuitive, giving, calm, connected and focused on relationships and partnerships. The use of both will be the difference between an average and an extraordinary human.

I love roadmaps and I love a How-To, so if you've reached the end of this chapter, I bet you're looking for something similar.

Find a chiropractic mentor. One that aligns with the way you want to practice and communicate and has excelled in something you want to experience.

Clusterbook. Fill your adjusting hours from the inside out and don't extend hours until that time slot is full. I recommend time studies if you're building your practice volume (or your business approach has changed) by having your CA track your time per adjustment.

Base your hours on your ideal patient. Are they working moms who can only come in the afternoon/evenings? Do you live in a rural region where people need to drive to get to you? Are you downtown so the majority of your practice are executive business people? Create your hours based on your niche or who you are looking to attract.

Always use your intuition when adjusting. Well, when doing anything, but allow the right brain to be activated through every adjustment.

Get reviews. Whether it's a product like Review Wave or an internal system, ask your patients to share their story.

Apps that we love:
Document creation: Google Docs, Google Forms
Team communication: Slack, Voxer
Project management: Asana
Team training: Loom, Zoom
Marketing graphics: Canva

Chiropractors are in the business of aligning the brain and the body for optimal function. It's time we do the same for our businesses. We know there is no one-size-fits-all plan for any patient, because the number of variables won't allow it. The same is true of your practice - you need a business plan tailored to YOU.

You can't build a business that thrives if it is simultaneously beating you down; its health is only as sustainable as its tie to your vitality. If we begin with an honest self-assessment, taking a solid inventory of our strengths and consciously working with our weaknesses, we can present ourselves with unwavering confidence. THAT is the spine of your practice. A team that aligns and complements that is the musculature that empowers the limbs of your business. Complement that solid structure with strong systems, appropriate delegation, respected leadership and a whole lotta heart and you'll quickly find yourself with a practice, life, team and family you are excited to nurture and serve.

Wisdom #26

Brian Kelly DC

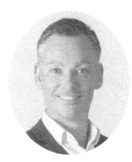

Brian Kelly has been a chiropractor for 28 years. He has been president of the NZ College of Chiropractic and in 2011 was president of Life Chiropractic College-West in California, the first non-American to lead a US Chiropractic college. He has also been president of the Australian Spinal Research Foundation and a board member for over 10 years.

Dr Kelly has led several trips to India where he has spoken to audiences of over a million people. He is the CAA (Vic) 2001 Chiropractor of the Year, the 2007 International Chiropractor of the Year awarded by Parker Seminars, the 2009 NZ Chiropractor of the Year and in 2014 he was nominated by his peers to be a Fellow of the International Chiropractors' Association. When not seeing patients, Brian spends time with his 3 children and plays in jazz bands.

How are you?

"How are you?" is a question we often ask our friends, family, or colleagues. As healthcare practitioners we are obliged to ask it of our patients. It is definitely a social norm that we all use.

The typical response is, "Yeah, good thanks", or "Been super busy", or even a "Not too bad".

But what the heck does that all mean and what are we really asking, or asking for?

We may ask the question to show interest in another human

being, and then hope they will ask us the same, so we can say how great things are, or what we have recently achieved. Some use it as an opportunity to vent, or to complain about their latest problem.

The question is infrequently posed to ascertain how a person *really* is, how they are *really feeling*, what is *really bothering them*, or even to enquire as to how we may help.

It is often great to ask the question, just to be a good listener. As we listen to someone and they talk through what is going on in their life, this itself can bring clarity to them. I'm sure we have all been on both sides of this.

I was recently chatting with a friend, a very good friend. We were talking on the phone and I asked him how he was doing. After the usual customary, "Yeah not bad mate", he then lowered his guard a little and said some of the things he had been up to. It was a dark place. Very dark. I said let's catch up for dinner soon. He agreed but had some family things going on, so the earliest we could meet was 10 days later.

Time passed and I texted to confirm dinner on the day. I did not hear back. Strange. The next morning, I phoned him and it went to voicemail. This was unusual. But within a couple of hours I had heard through friends and then had it confirmed that he had taken his own life. I remember vividly hearing the news. I was out cycling, and I was devastated. I was bawling on the side of the road. Truly heartbroken that someone who I was close to, shared intimate conversations with, conversations of meaning and vulnerability, had decided he could not go on with life.

Had I known, I would have done what...? I would have done whatever I could to ease the pain, the deep suffering and to try and walk in his shoes to offer help out of this very dark place.

"How are You?" In healthcare and in chiropractic it's a question that's asked not only on the initial visit, but on every visit. But what are we really asking?

When a patient replies with, "I'm doing great with my health/symptom/problem", do we breathe a sigh of relief and let it confirm that Chiropractic really works? If there is no great symptomatic change, or the patient is feeling an exacerbation of symptoms, do we feel concerned that we may be missing something? Or do we accept that healing can take time, and the body can and will go through some non-linear changes?

The question I really pose to chiropractors is, why are people actually coming to see us? And why do they often stay with us long after their initial complaint has resolved?

I had a patient recently who came in with severe pain. On his second visit I curiously asked how he was doing and he replied, "I'm still in pain, but I feel better". This is a profound statement. He was aware he was still injured, but there had been a shift in his body. Something had changed. If we were simply giving drugs to mask the symptoms, this would be an unlikely response.

As a healthcare practitioner you can set up your office to help create an environment of healing and love. When you do, people will come for something greater. They will come because it feels different being with you and your staff. They will feel a connection. It takes intention to create this. The clinic layout, the colours, your choice of music, reading material, ambience, and the mood and vibration of you and your staff.

When you create this environment, you will find people often arrive early, they stay late, and they often keep coming more frequently than you recommend. They may even comment to their friends, "I'm not sure why I go, I just go".

As a chiropractor, in addition to laying our hands on people, and the magic of human touch, we get to adjust the spine and perform specific, well-intentioned adjustments to remove nerve interference, and correct subluxations. This is a remarkable contribution to humanity.

A subluxation affects the biomechanics of the spine, alters nervous system function, and can have a myriad of negative effects on the function of the body, including immune function. My initial personal experience was as a 7-year-old when I went to the chiropractor following multiple bouts of tonsillitis.

The problem with subluxation, is that pain and symptoms are a poor indicator of whether you have one. You could have a sore back from hitting 200 golf balls and may not have a subluxation at all; or you could have an upper cervical subluxation for years manifesting as, say, multiple sclerosis, and have no spinal pain associated with it.

Back to how are you feeling.

If we have compromise or interference with the nervous system, the body and brain will not have optimal function. We now have some tools to measure this. Some tools are in the research lab and may include PET scans or fMRI scans. A lot of this has been published.

So why do people keep coming to the chiropractor, long after their symptoms have reduced, or they still have the same initial presenting complaint, say migraine headaches? Because there is a shift in the physiology in how their body is functioning, and they know innately or subjectively that getting adjusted is good for them. They keep coming for care because their life is different.

Are pain and suffering the same thing?

I don't believe they are. If you have a context on why you have symptoms or an injury, it is very possible to be in some level of pain but not be suffering.

But what is the opposite situation? The person who has little to no pain, but a spine that is causing major compromise to nerve and body function? Could it lead to mental health issues, could it affect sleep, immune function, could it affect organ function? Could it lower the vibration of someone's life so life is not what it could be?

Can you have no spinal symptoms and still have reduced function in the body from altered spinal mechanics and therefore nerve function? Not only can you, but I would also contend that it happens every time. We have all seen the nerve charts that show spinal pain is only 10% of the nerve story, so we do know that feeling does not relate to function.

We could eat the highest quality organic food, exercise daily, meditate and live a life of purpose, but if you don't have a sound functioning nerve system function, you are not getting the most out of life.

So how are you?

Yes, it's a social norm, a clinical question to breathe a sigh of relief that the person is getting what they came for, or a box you tick for an insurance case, but what is your real purpose in Chiropractic? What service are you really offering your community?

When I asked my friend how he was doing, he gave me a big clue. I should have driven over and seen him straight away. Was he in pain? Maybe not physical pain but on many deep levels he was suffering tremendously. And if any of us who knew him knew that, we would have done more. We would have done whatever it takes.

So, I urge my colleagues to think about what their higher purpose in Chiropractic is and what service we are really offering humanity. Given that most subluxations cause no pain or symptoms, then we are adjusting people for a very different purpose.

Some of the strategies you might employ could be:

Keep doing the things you do that help create the best version of yourself.

See the flowers and not the weeds. What we focus on grows. Complaining won't change too much in your life, but may bring more of what you are complaining about.

When you ask someone, "How are you?", listen to what they are really saying, and maybe also the unsaid.

And finally, when someone asks, "How are you?", open your heart. Be human.

David Fletcher DC, FRCCS(C)

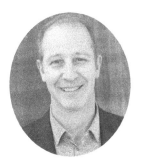

As chiropractic moves further into the neuroAge, David is recognised as one of the leading champions of this transitional shift as the innovator of the INSiGHT scanning technologies. His passion for teaching success-based, principled strategies coupled with the certainty that experience brings, is a potent and inspiring message for today's Chiropractic.

An accomplished communicator, a Fellow in the Chiropractic Sport Sciences and owner/President of CLA, David's message helps bridge the widening gap within the profession by blending the neurosciences with practical solutions for everyday practitioners.

The truth of the matter

"When men differ... both sides ought equally to have the advantage of being heard by the public... for when Truth and Error have fair play, the former is always an overmatch for the latter."

Benjamin Franklin

The "truth of the matter" is a phrase that is commonly used to emphasise a particular point of view. It accentuates facts being discussed, which are not widely known or recognised, or could even be a secret.

The truth of the matter is that Chiropractic is the answer to an ailing society and a troubled world.

From its humblest beginnings, using an evidence-informed approach, the chiropractic pioneers boldly asserted that the tone of the nervous system was instrumental, if not paramount, in the expression of the human experience and condition. They posited that this tone could be altered by the instantaneous or cumulative effects of stressors originating from either "traumas, toxins or thoughts". Alongside this daring assertion, they codified a set of deductive and inductively reasoned principles that acted as guides to understand the interplay between universal forces, matter, intelligent design and the expression of life itself. How audacious!

The truth of the matter is that Chiropractic is founded on principles that extend far beyond the boundaries of human health and symptoms.

The 33 Principles, as they are fondly referred to, begin with a clarifying statement known as the Major Premise. Its first 4 words instantly define the distinctiveness of chiropractic philosophy and its intended place in affecting, understanding and improving the human condition.

The Major Premise (Principle #1): *A Universal Intelligence is in all matter and continually gives to it all its properties and actions, thus maintaining it in existence.*

Principle #1 asserts that the existence of all matter, including the human body and its complexity of functional parts, is imbued with a universal intelligence thereby establishing an intelligent design. By framing the entire premise for chiropractic's existence on this statement, a profession was created to exemplify the power of addressing health and healing from the inside-out. In today's vernacular, Chiropractic can be described as taking a salutogenic approach rather than a pathogenic one. Salutogenesis, as defined by Antonofsky, is a stress-resource based approach that examines the factors which promote physical and mental well-being rather than being focused on the management of disease.

The genius of the 33 Principles beginning with a statement of fact that all matter exists because of Universal Intelligence, sets the stage for an examination of forces that interfere with the expression of this perfection. With this philosophical construct in place, well-being and health need no longer be defined by pathology and symptoms but rather as a subset of an intelligent design striving to maximise its expression and potential. If unlimited potential, within the limitations of matter, is the starting point for the human journey, the focus of Chiropractic can then be shifted towards determining and addressing obstructions to the expression of life.

The truth of the matter is that for life to be established and maintained, there must be a coherent triunity between Intelligence, Force and Matter.

The framer of the 33 Principles, Ralph W Stephenson DC, understood the necessity of bringing the chiropractic meaning of life forward in the earliest principles and then creating a logical formula to show how intelligence and matter could coordinate (Principle #2). However, to establish his argument that the expression of life was the ultimate outcome, Stephenson needed to add a third element to bind together the first 2 elements. To vivify Matter, Force must be present, thereby creating a triunity that delivers life as an outcome (Principles #8, 9, 10). The Triune of Life brings together Intelligence, Force and Matter so that a chiropractor can now focus on what is directly changeable, while expecting an outcome in line with the expression of a coherent life (Principles #4, 5). Force interacts with matter by creating motion and the function of intelligence is to create force. This sets up the obvious outcome which is a dynamic confluence known as intelligent life. What is most exciting within this formulaic construct is the ability for an outside force to be introduced with the intent of removing interference patterns, thereby creating greater coherence between intelligence and matter. Remember, when intelligence organises and organised matter remains wildly efficient, this supports the expression of full potential. A chiropractic adjustment (force) delivered with the intent of reducing or interrupting interference patterns as demonstrated by lost motion, can be aligned with the expectation of manifesting greater life expression (Principle #15).

But what motion are we observing and measuring? Is it the entire body's mobility, mobility of spinal parts or the transmission of more subtle forces that coordinate motion and function within the human system? For force to be effective it must be distributable and uninterrupted so that intelligence can always be present, right down to the most intricate intracellular and quantum levels. The most complex and omnipresent transmission system tasked with control over all other systems is the central nervous system (Principle #29). Whether synaptic or non-synaptic, the nervous system distributes the uninterrupted messages of force and intelligence to all matter within the human body. The nervous system holds the key to a chiropractor's interactive art and skills, based upon the science and the philosophy of life expression.

The truth of the matter is that the tone of the nervous system is directly influenced by a chiropractic adjustment.

"Life is the expression of tone". So said DD Palmer as he originated his conceptual framework for Chiropractic's existence. He described tone as the normal degree of nerve tension. "Consequently, the cause of disease is any variation of tone; nerves too tense or too slack."

In today's clinical conversations, tone is used when describing certain neurological activity. Vagal tone refers to "the continual baseline parasympathetic action that the vagus nerve exerts." This baseline of tonality forms the foundation for the theoretical development of the subluxation and the value and purpose of a chiropractic adjustment. The natural, homeo-dynamic responsiveness exerts an "ideal" tone, allowing function and adaptability to operate within a range of ease. Forces applied beyond these innate, adaptive boundaries cause a reaction to occur (Principle #17). As such, the tone or tension within the responding nervous system becomes altered. The tensegrity of the affected organs and cells must be maintained at the baseline level of tonal response to function optimally. Should the interference patterns become persistent, the law of adaptability within intelligent systems dictates that a new responsive, habituated baseline be established (Principle #6, 24).

This new normal is representative of the affected adaptation and as such is inefficient, compared to the optimal performance of an unaltered pattern. Habituation of the interference to the tone of the nervous system is surmised within the chiropractic cosmology to be the basis of disease (Principle #30). The restoration of normal function is attributable to the removal or correction of the interference. Subluxations are the manifestation of the adaptive responses and are present when the interference to transmission is present and persistent (Principle #6, 31).

The truth of the matter is that subluxations are identifiable and measurable.

The central nervous system is universally involved in all disease. The tone of the nervous system affects the transmission of adaptive responses, thereby altering the intelligent expression of the matter (body) as it reacts to the primal forces of nature and the demands of exogenous and emotional stressors. By measuring the capability and ranges of transmission within the functional nervous system, a chiropractor can deduce whether the subluxation is present and to what degree it is causing interference.

Two standardised metrics can be evaluated when assessing neural tone. The amplitude and symmetry of the neural signalling can be measured using validated and reproducible instrumentation. Electromyography (EMG) testing shows us the performance within the motor nervous system while thermography and heart rate variability are recognised for identifying dysautonomia. Inclinometry quantifies dyskinesia. When applied with the intent of observing noxious patterns while being compared to normative, well-adjusted cohorts, the tonality of the nervous system can be related to the presence of vertebral subluxations. As function of the neural transmission is altered, there is the probability that adaptability will wane. Compensation in function, motion, structure, and performance are sequential with the final injustice being the dimming of an individual's potential.

The truth of the matter is that Chiropractic works.

The keen observation and measurement by a chiropractor, operating through the lens of the 33 Principles, confirms the presence of vertebral subluxations. By accepting and understanding the devastating toll that vertebral subluxations have on the expression of human health and potential, chiropractors can become the beacon for an ailing society and troubled world. The boldness of the Chiropractic, with its philosophical construct, scientific models and evidence-informed approach to clinical application, is necessary now, more than ever. As stressors from the ever present "thoughts, traumas and toxins" overtake an ill-informed public, the simplicity and elegance of Chiropractic's art, philosophy and applied sciences offer a hopeful future where the truth matters more than the rhetoric.

Fred H Barge DC, a legendary scribe within Chiropractic, sums up the universality and the simplicity of Chiropractic's philosophy, application and genius:

"There is but one cause in disease, the bodies inability to comprehend itself and/or its environment.
There is but one cure in disease, the body's ability to heal itself.
And there is only one thing any doctor can do for a patient.
And that is to remove an obstruction to healing, thus, facilitating it."

Wisdom #27

Larry Markson DC

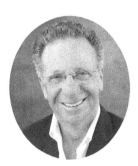

Dr. Larry Markson has been a Personal Empowerment, Success and Prosperity Coach to over 28,000 chiropractors for the past 40 years. He has devoted his professional life to assisting others in transforming their inner dialogs, concepts, visions, actions and feelings until they are able to create a life of fulfilment and significance. Larry has been a Chiropractor for 59 years and is in his fifth decade of sharing the secrets of personal & business growth, inner success and unlimited attraction power with audiences nationwide. His new creation is the Chiro-Cabin, a 1½ day Personal and Professional Retreat that guides Chiropractors, their Associate doctors and entire staff down a path that leads to Abundant Health, Wonderful Relationships, a Thriving Practice and Financial Freedom.

It is Essential & It is Right

In his classic, *A Tale of Two Cities, Charles Dickens wrote:* "It was the best of times and it was the worst of times. It was the age of wisdom and it was the age of foolishness. It was the epic of belief and it was the epic of incredulity. It was the season of light and it was the season of darkness. It was the spring of hope and it was the winter of despair. We had everything before us, we had nothing before us. We were all going direct to heaven or we were all going the other way."

That was in 1789. In 1895, now 125 years ago, it was the story of the chiropractors who first began to put forth our chiropractic principles. That incredible wisdom will finally spread around the world or it will remain the same; a secret. Nothing changes, yet everything must change – starting right now!

Nation upon nation is clamouring for change in just about everything, but particularly in their healthcare delivery systems and I have learned over the years, what the people want, they eventually get.

My purpose is to attempt to place in perspective the tremendous metamorphosis that is happening, how our profession is positioned now, and how this relentless evolution in healthcare will be affecting our entire future.

Is this the age of great opportunity that we so loosely speak about or is it the age of great fear? Is it the age to capitulate or is it the age to stand and fight for this precious principle of ours?

If our goal is to earn the public's trust and respect, and to ensure our role in the future, we must all must make some essential corrections in this great profession.

Let me spell out some examples.

It is essential that ALL chiropractic colleges including the brand new Scottish College of Chiropractic teach chiropractic principle as part of their core curriculum. From my point of view, indeed from every point of view, it is this very philosophy that makes us unique and so vital and necessary, in an era when other healthcare disciplines are no longer trusted.

It is essential that our doctors have the ability to use mass media to articulate our principles and our purpose to the public at large; and do so in a way that Mr & Mrs Public can clearly understand and comprehend what we are really all about.

It is essential that we as a profession develop a sensible and sane procedural protocol so our image can adapt, modify, change and modernise, so we can start to flourish rather than be held back by being labelled as a fragmented profession.

It is essential to make a unified and concerted effort for unity within our entire profession, especially with regard to a massive effort at educating the public about the short and long-term benefits derived from having a nervous system that works properly, thanks to the talent and skill of a qualified and competent chiropractor.

It is essential that our practitioners have fundamental practice management skills so they can gracefully transfer from student, to practitioner, to ultra-successful natural healthcare facilitators.

It is essential that low self-esteem DCs be prevented from hurting all of us by using immoral, unethical and/or dishonest methods of practice, just because they believe that's the only way they can survive.

It is essential that we begin to police our own profession, to monitor and end true over-utilisation of visits, fraudulent billing practices, bait-and-switch techniques, insurance fraud, low-class advertising, give-it-away-free schemes and/or any other procedure or tactic that causes us to lose in the long run.

We must have integrity that comes from within. It is not enough to be well behaved just because regulatory agencies threaten censure of penalty and legislatures threaten us with restrictions.

It is essential to discourage DCs from becoming the shills of unscrupulous attorneys, the lackeys of insurance companies and the servants of the almighty buck! This is a time for Chiropractic to grow and glow, not a time for sleaze!

Let's reinforce and respond to those things that make

Chiropractic a true beacon for outstanding natural healthcare

As a personal and practice development coach for the past 40 years, I am calling for a central core of chiropractic strength that emphasizes what is RIGHT about Chiropractic. For example:

It is right that DCs and their offices provide a first class, state-of-the-art, healing art option to the people of their communities.

It is right that DCs have offices that project the professionalism of a great profession, and that they are constructed in such a manner as to send notice that this is a place of natural and holistic healing, representative of the finest in healthcare delivery.

It is right that DCs have professional expertise, procedural efficiency, business acumen and personality traits geared for success.

It is right, yes, very right, that DCs and CAs are constantly trained to do empowering daily affirmations, set and achieve worthy goals and strive for high standards of excellence.

It is right that DCs learn to have a compassion to serve vs. just a compulsion to survive, and that they have honest fees, ethical procedures, respect for themselves and love for our profession.

It is right that DCs protect their families against catastrophe by securing malpractice and other essential insurance.

It is right that chiropractic assistants are trained to paraprofessional status and encouraged to keep learning more so they can better contribute to a patient's healthcare.

It is right that DCs learn to build strong and positive self-images and to become leaders in their offices and in their communities, as well.

All of the above is right and essential if you want to build the practices of your dreams while you enjoy the happiest, healthiest and most prosperous lifestyles you can imagine.

Chiropractic in A Changing Healthcare Environment

In my opinion, one single factor is going to reshape healthcare in the next few years. Unfortunately, it will not be the quality of care; it will not be universal access; and it will have nothing to do with high technology. That one driving factor will be economics!

Government and the marketplace will continuously try to reduce the cost of healthcare. However, despite your initial negative reaction, this will eventually create a tremendous opportunity for the chiropractic profession.

Here's why. All the research of the past decade proves that medicine is ponderous, uncaring and costly, and this same research shows Chiropractic to be not only clinically effective, but cost effective and the home run hitter in patient satisfaction. We ARE the natural choice when the policy makers look for ways to solve the healthcare disaster.

Sadly, nothing will happen unless this profession has a strong, coherent strategy to make sure that it happens. That strategy must come from a united front and from one unified approach. The time has come to stop circling the wagons and shooting in at ourselves. The target is outside and the victory comes from us singing one song to the legislative bodies and one patient education song to every man, woman and child... around the world. Then we will see the greatness of this profession!

Ramneek S. Bhogal DC, DABI

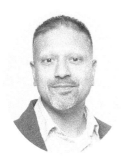

A 2002 Palmer graduate, Ramneek has served the profession through 20 years of teaching, having recently retired as Professor and Head of Technique at Life West. He was extremely active within student leadership organisations and his passion continues in private practice where his expertise and experience allows him to help patients labelled as "complex cases."

He is published in JMPT, having researched methodologies to measure forces produced by chiropractic techniques. He also was published in the Journal of Clinical Chiropractic Pediatrics and is himself a peer reviewer for other journals and often speaks at national conferences.

What I have learned

There I stood, in front of a classroom of my peers and some students. It was a mixed seminar peppered with vitalists and mechanists and just like the hundreds of seminars and classes I have taught in my 20 years of education, I was a cool mixture of anxious and excited. In the final moments of preparation, I had decided to veer from my scripted lecture and I felt a little uneasy about it. It was 2017 and an age-old topic had reared its toxic head, again.

The chiropractic profession was bantering again about whether the word "subluxation" had a place in chiropractic education. That perhaps it had a better place in the annals of history, to be discussed as a lost theory. My mind was set, the conversation was going to take place and I wanted usher in the idea of the power of the adjustment and the gravity of the vertebral subluxation complex. Yet somehow, I had to weave it elegantly into a diagnosis lecture pertaining to congenital cardiac abnormalities. This life had prepared me well.

I arrived at chiropractic college in Davenport, Iowa in 1998 and I can proudly say I was the product of educators like Virgil Strang, Fred Barge, and Bruce Lipton. I was also blessed with the company of greats like Sid Williams, Bud Crowder, and Reggie Gold. With that same sense of pride, I will share with you that, more importantly, the words of those great philosophers were peals of bells that forged my understanding of Chiropractic for the next 20 years in both clinical practice and in chiropractic education. As I grew as a clinician and as I made my way to the rank of professor, the wisdom and truth in their words took shape. So, I stood in front of that crowd in 2017 with the voices of giants in my head, heart, and hands.

"What is the cause of dis-ease?", I asked this chiropractic smorgasbord of 150 attendees. At first, no one responded. I used more force and repeated myself again and again until they all understood that I was serious. Finally, there were mumblings and I could make out that the majority were answering, "The subluxation". I accepted their group answer, for now, and proceeded. Next, I went on to share the reality behind the chiropractic ideology of "one cause, one cure". It must be understood that the cause of dis-ease is not the subluxation, but rather, the failure to adapt to stimulus. Principle #21 speaks to the Mission of Innate Intelligence and the premise that innate's mission is to maintain the body in active organisation. Some may prefer the term homeostasis.

In either case, this task is accomplished through adaptability.

This idea of adaptation is the body's inherent biological ability to redirect and negotiate, for the better, in response to varying stimuli in one's environment. So why are we so attached to the idea of the subluxation? Let me suggest to you that the subluxation results in the physical perception of dis-ease.

The neuro-musculo-skeletal dysregulation that is lived by the patient as loss of quality of life through impaired function or pain. This has made the subluxation the centre point of "cause". Let me be so bold as to state that perhaps we need to think of two varieties of "cause". Let us start by understanding that a compromised capacity to adapt to stimuli brings the subluxation into existence. We fail to adapt to, or negotiate, the thoughts, traumas, and toxins in our lives and, as such, a subluxation is birthed into reality. If we carry this notion forwards, we can now consider the second "cause".

This is the aforementioned physical perception of the subluxation complex. All the symptoms that a clinician must navigate with the patient. Simply put, the subluxation causes the patient to have symptoms.

This brings us to this question about "one cure". Again, I asked the crowd for their thoughts and the overwhelming response was "the chiropractic adjustment". Logically if the "cause" is the subluxation then the "cure" must be the adjustment? As I pivoted the conversation, I proposed the notion that the "cure" is the body's inherent ability to heal itself, and not the adjustment. While the cure is unleashed by the adjustment, it isn't the adjustment that does the curing, it merely removes the inference that hinders the body's ability to cure itself.

So, if the "cause" is the compromised capacity to adapt

and the "cure" is the body's ability to heal itself, what does this mean for the chiropractor? Read on.

I understand and respect that innate intelligence is an organised expression of universal intelligence and that it is expressed through a physical body with limitations. In my infancy of philosophical growth, my emphatic understanding revolved around this concept of "expression". I was driven by the misguided fact that all I needed to do was to adjust my patients. But in this fool's wisdom, I realised that my patients were dependent upon me and the adjustment I could deliver. I, in fact, became a part of the limitation.

As I matured in my thinking and as I matured as a chiropractor, I began to appreciate the limitations of matter as a reality in clinical conversation and patient education. The quintessential question became, "to what does the patient fail to adapt and can that be changed?". I placed an emphasis on not only the "3 T's" of thoughts, traumas, and toxins, but I added another "T". Threshold. My paradigm shifted slightly and my narrative changed dramatically with my patients. The conversation turned to what components of the "3 T's" was the patient navigating and being challenged with. In essence, what was each individual's threshold with the stimuli to which they failed to adapt. Basically, how much could they handle, before they faltered into a subluxated state? It was paramount to now mitigate these "T's" so as to effectuate a better threshold. The clinical reality manifested as patients who were maintaining better neuro-musclo-skeletal health in between care appointments and the physical perceptions of the subluxation began to diminish.

These same patients realised a better quality of life, robust with better function and well-being overall. Chiropractic care turned from intervention to prevention. My practice had evolved and was oscillating around a new axis.

Now, 20 years' practice and education leave it clear and critical to me, that as a profession, we must be as neurologically informed as possible when detecting the vertebral subluxation complex with due diligence exercised in neurological, muscular, and skeletal systems. To also employ the use of objective measurement wherever and whenever possible to quantify the subluxation.

As a past Department Head of Technique I also firmly believe that adjusting techniques are not methodologies etched in stone to be prescriptive for all, but rather, are tools to be utilised for the job at hand. That job is dictated by the patient's presentation. When asked by so many in my career, "Dr Bhogal, what technique do you practice?", my steadfast answer is, "Give me a patient to evaluate and then I will tell you." All techniques should be exercised with discipline however, once chosen as the best tool for the subluxation at hand.

I close with the notion that our profession is in need, now more than ever, of discipline and adherence to being neurologically informed and driven by a desire to find the cause. As you go forth to serve, please guard this notion well.

Wisdom#28

Jonathan M P Howat DC, DICS, FICS, FRCC (paed), FRCC (cranio), FEAC (cranio)

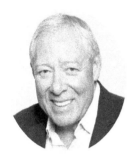

Jonathan graduated from the Palmer College of Chiropractic in 1970, then returned to his home in Rhodesia to practice with his father David P Howat (graduate from the Palmer School of Chiropractic in 1937). In 1975 he was involved in chiropractic legislation for Rhodesia. He emigrated to the UK in 1984 and two years later, started SOTO Europe, a teaching organisation using SOT protocols which is still being taught today.

Over the last 30 years, Jonathan has taught SOT and CFD in Japan, Brazil, Chile, Australia, South Africa, the USA, Hong Kong, Singapore, Germany, Italy, Holland, France, Switzerland, Sweden and the UK.

In 2019 he founded and developed the Howat Institute of Cranio Fascial Dynamics teaching the 'Howat 8 Step Protocols' for brain injury and brain drainage. He has various publications to his name and since 1985 has been clinical director of the Oxford Chiropractic Clinic.

Chiropractic: Traumatic brain injury and brain damage

After many years of observing patients and their posture, facial configurations and jaw deviation, it has become clear that the cranial reciprocal tension membrane (RTM) system, consisting of:

· The falx cerebri

- The tentorium cerebellum
- The falx cerebellum
- The diaphragma selli

has a direct effect on the way the brain moves and how its drainage pattern influences homeostasis. The venous sinus system is totally encapsulated by the dural membrane and is part of the meningeal dura, which covers the brain surface, and the endosteal layer – covering the internal cranial bone surfaces, respectively. The venous sinus system is responsible for draining the brain of venous blood which it does primarily through the superior sagittal and inferior sagittal sinuses, being the 2 most significant vessels.

According to Gray's Anatomy, the superior sagittal sinus drains into the right transvers sinus, the right sigmoid sinus and then into the right internal jugular vein. The inferior sagittal sinus drains into the left transverse sinus, the left sigmoid sinus and then into the left internal jugular vein. The drainage on the right side has bigger vessels than on the left, and according to research, larger volumes of venous blood are drained from the right side than from the left. The volume of venous blood that is drained from these vessels causes a haemodynamic flow from right to left, creating a minute counter-clockwise movement of the brain.

As a result of this haemodynamic force, the cranial membranes also move in a counter-clockwise direction producing a cranio-fascial torsion which then influences the infant cranium. The foetus demonstrates venous drainage early on in its development, so this haemodynamic force is in place before the infant birth and so appears before the cranial plates evolve.

When the infant cranium grows after birth, the earlier influence of haemodynamic forces changes the shape of the cranium as it develops into the adult form. The cranium becomes more oblong with a right frontal area more expansive than the left, and a left occipital area more expansive than the right. The sphenoid bone – the central bone of the cranium – has the right greater wing in a superior anterior attitude (presenting a larger ocular orbit and a pronounced right eye) relative to the left greater wing which appears in an inferior posterior attitude (presenting a smaller ocular orbit and a retracted left eye). This torsioned sphenoid also effects the diaphragma selli, the tentorium cerebellum and the tentorial incisura, of the cranial membrane system.

The cranio-fascial torsion in the brain and the resultant drainage process must, from a haemodynamic standpoint, also indicate that the heart (the pump) and the liver (the filter) being placed off-centre in the body, will also create a haemodynamic thrust through the entire arterial venous system for homeostasis to exist. Like rifling in a gun to propel the bullet and to create momentum in its striking ability, the haemodynamic thrust is required to remove residue within the vascular system in order to eliminate a build-up of superfluous material in those vessels.

Why is this subject so important to understand and what is its significance in brain function restoration? The cranio-fascial torque of the brain influences arterial inflow; the circle of Willis (internal carotid and vertebral arteries), the venous sinus system (brain drainage), the ventricular system (brain core) and cranio-dental aspects are all factors which need to be understood in order to correct the cranium.

Brain Drainage

The brain is an irrigation system; equal volumes of blood into the brain and equal volumes out of the brain. The venous sinus system is totally encapsulated by the dural membrane and is responsible for draining the brain of venous blood, which it does primarily through the superior sagittal and inferior sagittal sinuses, being the 2 most significant vessels.

This venous blood then flows through the superior sagittal sinus towards the confluence of the sinuses, where it diverts into the right transverse sinus, the right sigmoid sinus into the right internal jugular vein which then passes through the right jugular foramen. These sinuses are encapsulated by the tentorium cerebellum at the transverse groove of the occiput, and are detrimentally influenced by cranio fascial torque. This represents the anterior superior drainage of the brain.

The inferior sagittal sinus encapsulated by the inferior border of the falx cerebri, collects venous blood from the internal cerebral vein, the basil vein and the Great vein of Galen before joining the straight sinus anteriorly at the junction of the falx cerebri and the falx cerebelli which the joins posteriorly at the confluence of the sinuses. It then drains into the left transverse sinus, the left sigmoid sinus and the left internal jugular vein exiting through the left jugular foramen; separate pathways. This represents the anterior inferior drainage of the brain.

The cavernous sinuses drain into the superior and inferior petrosal sinuses, encapsulated by the tentorium cerebellum along the petrous portion of the temporal bone and drains into the sigmoid sinus before exiting through the internal jugular vein.

The basilar venous plexus partially drains the cavernous and inter-cavernous sinuses into the anterior, lateral and posterior vertebral venous plexus, situated around the ring of the foramen magnum and then into the sub-occipital cavernous sinus.

This vast and complex venous drainage allows the intracranial pressure to be controlled as well as cooling the incoming arterial flow, by adjusting the flow and intensity through this grid to control homeostasis.

The ventricular system

The ventricular system is the core of the brain and the extension of the spinal cord. The roof of the two lateral ventricles is the corpus callosum, also supporting the supracallosal gyrus and the cingulate gyrus; responsible for retrieval and processing and disseminating data from the rest of the brain.

The lateral inferior borders of the lateral ventricles is supported by the caudate nucleus – learning and processing memories and recall.

The central part of the lateral ventricles is supported by the fornix - memory recall and hippocampus processing - part of the limbic system.

The third ventricle is surrounded and supported by the thalamus and hypothalamus – the junction boxes of the brain, disseminating information from the cortex to the spinal cord and vice versa.

The fourth ventricle is supported anteriorly by the pons and cerebral peduncles - communication from the cortex to the pons, laterally by the cerebellar peduncle - information to and from midbrain, pons and cerebellum, and posteriorly by the cerebellum.

This central core area is the communication centre of the

brain, surrounded by neurological pathways and conduits propagating neurological information around the brain and central nervous system. The ventricular system is also invested in the frontal parietal, temporal and occipital lobes of the brain, storage houses from which the brain core retrieves vital information.

Trauma

Brain trauma of any magnitude is exemplified by a change in the cranial membrane system.

The counter-clockwise motion of the brain produces a benign counter-clockwise torque of the cranium - this is normal and asymmetric and has no clinical presentation. However, when trauma is introduced, the benign asymmetry becomes a traumatic asymmetric torque. This torque is more emphasised and manifests clinical changes – neurologically, physically and from a fascial stand-point. The traumatic force can be a diaschisis force, acting in the same direction as the counter-clockwise torque, or a necrotic force which is clockwise and in the opposite direction to the original asymmetric counter-clockwise torque, and consequently more devastating to the brain stem.

Birth trauma with forceps intervention will disrupt the atlanto-occipital junction putting immense pressure onto the vertebral arteries as they penetrate the atlanto-occipital membrane.

Whiplash trauma will damage the cervical spine, creating early degenerative changes to ligaments, muscles and possibly the intervertebral discs, certainly, to the mid and lower cervical spine. This sort of trauma has a direct affect on the vertebral arteries, resulting in possible tearing and bleeding with resultant potential blockage of the vessels.

Subluxations of the atlas and axis (C2) will distort the atlanto-occipital membrane, causing a narrowing and stretching of the vessels, changing arterial flow into the basilar artery and the posterior aspect of the circle of Willis. This in turn over the years gives rise to blockages and would possibly account for the 15% of congenital aneurysms found in the posterior circulation of the brain.

But, possibly trauma to the body, neck and head will have its most adverse effect on the ventricular system; the core brain components. Changing pathways and conduits will potentially have the most devastating impact on neurological communications and a lifelong affect on brain function.

Cranio fascial dynamics

Cranio fascial dynamics are specific intra-oral cranial adjustments designed to address the mobility of the cervical spine and reduce cranio fascial torque in the membrane system, in order to re-establish normal homeostasis. This is the first step in trying to combat the damage delivered through physical trauma sustained throughout life to the central nervous system. This is a physical correction. Cranio fascial torque is a fact of life and unless removed, all other traumas compact, and become secondary and tertiary to the stability of the brain and spinal cord. These are the problems The Howat 8 Step Protocols are designed to deal with.

Cranio Fascial Dynamics (CFD) is designed to access the type of trauma to the brain and spinal cord - primarily the 80% of the central nervous system in the cranium - using neurological, fascial and physical indicators around the body and the cranium. They address any traumatic forces and attempt to reverse those forces. Trauma of any sort will produce a torque effect, either clockwise or counter-clockwise, on the brain core. Each subsequent trauma throughout life is superimposed on the haemodynamic counter-clockwise motion of the brain generated in utero. This is a primary issue, thereby creating secondary and tertiary issues, which become the domain of chiropractic practice. Chiropractic must address the cranial torque issue, reinstate neurological pathways and reduce cranio fascial torque. This is our legacy laid down by the forefathers of our profession, DD and BJ and many, many others; to remove neurological interference. We have to claim what is justifiably part of Chiropractic; the philosophy, science and art. No one is addressing brain trauma and brain drainage. We ignore this area at our professional peril.

Paul McCrossin DC B.App.Sci (Chiro)

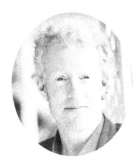

Paul has lived in the UK since 1998 and has established himself as an influential leader in the UK profession through his involvement in the United Chiropractic Association, of which he is now the President. The winner of the UCA Chiropractor of the Year Award in 2010, Paul also heads the peer & ethics committee, which allows him to fulfil his passion for helping other chiropractors in the UK to practice safely and ethically.

Paul has a special interest in how Chiropractic can help mothers throughout pregnancy and in the important role of chiropractic care in babies and children. He is married to Charlotte and they have two sons. In his free time, Paul is a keen endurance athlete and cyclist who has completed the Paris Brest Paris (a mere 1200km meander across France!) twice.

Be Yourself

I was humbled to be asked to contribute a chapter to a book, the proceeds of which are entirely to support such an important project for the chiropractic profession as the Scotland College of Chiropractic. It was even more poignant in that the profession lost a great chiropractor, leader, researcher and educator in Dr Dave Russell BSc(psych), BSc(chiro) who was soon to be the first college president. He was larger than life and had the personality and laugh to match.

Life can be full of clichés and such statements are often seen in a negative way, as they are overused. At one point however they commenced as inspired statements, and the principles behind them may be just as relevant. Dave used to say that "Chiropractic is a big **** deal", in his upfront way and he applied his curiosity as to how care impacted on the individual. If Chiropractic widely being a big deal becomes cliché, I don't see that as a negative eventuality, as it is what he and many of us would like to see.

I became a Chiropractor as it made sense to me. I was interested in health and not so much by treating symptoms using medication, rather by enhancing function in a physical sense. I would have wanted to be a surgeon if I was to study medicine. My career adviser in Australia, a Brit and ultra-marathon runner, suggested I look at Chiropractic. My thought, even at that age, was, don't they "just fix backs?" Now, once I investigated further and read that chiropractors focus on the spine, its function and the effects on the nervous system and health, it just made sense to me. So, I started getting checked and adjusted at that point, despite not having symptoms. At the time I thought it random chance that I came across Chiropractic, however on reflection I feel that I had a number of experiences that directed me to becoming a chiropractor.

I recall going along with a childhood friend on his visit to the chiropractor when I was in primary school. His mother was taking him, not because he had a specific injury or back complaint. I remember sitting in the reception room reading a pamphlet about subluxation and the spine and thinking I would like to be able to see a chiropractor. This particular chiropractor eventually became the President of the Chiropractors Association of Australia, as it was then known.

After deciding to study Chiropractic, I recall speaking with a family friend who was a long-time friend of my father, with whom he studied pharmacy in New Zealand. He ridiculed my decision, saying that he'd had a former mechanic speak at his rotary group about doing a weekend course to become a chiropractor. Clearly misinformed! While that was confronting, what surprised me was my father's searching questions on his knowledge of what chiropractic practice entails and the degree of study required to get a qualification. This was out of character for my father to be critical of a long-time friend and to unpick his bigoted opinion, particularly in front of his son. When I asked him about it, he told me his mother had taken him to Cyril Phelps, one of the first chiropractors in New Zealand, as a teenager because of scoliosis. This was news to me.

We all have those experiences where life seems to take a predetermined path, however I think that part of that is because we are drawn to and make decisions which are congruent with our values. Being aware of your own values and more importantly in practice, those of your practice members, is key for a successful and enjoyable practice.

We have all experienced the situation where we see a person who we know can literally have their quality of life changed by chiropractic care, yet they choose not to and instead opt to stay on a path that is not serving them or their health in the long term. It is frustrating and we have that internal dialogue, "Why don't they see what I see?" or to coin another cliché, "If people knew what you knew, they would do what you do." Some of the most passionate people I know are chiropractors and sometimes this passion and enthusiasm for what we do is blinding, ultimately meaning that we can be some of the worst communicators. So even if people know what you know it does not mean they will do what you do, as they don't place the same value on what you know. Health and the promotion of health may be of high value to many of us, however it is not always the case for those we see. It is rare to find a smoker who is unaware that it is harmful for them, yet they choose to continue, as what smoking brings to them is more important than the risk of long-term health effects. Why is the healthcare expenditure in the Western world so skewed in the direction of treating symptoms and disease and more specifically lifestyle-related diseases such as diabetes, cardiovascular disease and many cancers? It is because many value or place more importance on other things, such as their social life or career, than making the choices that will promote health in the long term. It goes beyond a choice between pleasure and pain.

It is simplistic to say that people's behaviours just revolve around either avoiding pain or seeking pleasure. It is true, however it is more nuanced. People will spend their time, and more importantly money, on what is important to them, and examining that will give a great clue as to what they value and what we as individuals value. These behaviours on a global scale may promote or erode their health in the long term. The NHS in England has a long-term plan to focus on the prevention of disease that, rather than just earlier detection, tries to prevent it in the first place. This centres on smoking, alcohol dependency, obesity and antimicrobial resistance. The difficulty for public health is that while awareness and education are very important, it is difficult to change behaviour by telling people what to do. It is not as successful in effecting change as connecting with the person and understanding what they are about. We as chiropractors have that opportunity, due to our model of care, which often involves developing relationships with people over time. A "wellness" model in the true sense of the word, not in the context of just having a regular adjustment but influencing change in behaviour to promote health, with a component being the function of the spine and nervous system.

One of the key things I have learnt in practice is that you cannot value someone's health more than they do, or place a value on health for them; only they can do that. Generally, people consult us because they are in pain, regardless of our viewpoint on who can benefit from care and when. They have a problem and they want it fixed. We have to establish what are symptoms making more difficult or preventing them doing that they value most, even before we think of the cause. In my experience many of the issues that result in people seeing a chiropractor are chronic, that is, they have had them for months or years. So, I ask, "Why now?" What has prompted them to do something now and generally it is because it has got to a point that it is affecting them on a level where it affects something they value.

Being able to connect on a humanistic level and focus on them as a person, their values, and not just the diagnosis or cause of their problem or symptoms is the core of a successful and enjoyable practice. At an undergraduate level we get very good at breaking down and reducing a person to a list of diagnoses, differentials and syndromes. Of course we need to know this, however, ultimately the person in front of us does not want to hear a lot of medical terminology. They want to know can you help reduce their limitations to help them to have better quality time with their family, play sport, socialise, be a better mother or father, earn money, prolong or enjoy their career more, to name a few. Early in my career, practice management was formulaic about "scripting" with chiropractors trying to be a copy of someone else which is one-sided and does not build understanding and connection.

Effective communication is a core component of successful and safe practice. In my years of helping chiropractors prevent and manage complaints from patients or to the regulator, the most common factor is poor or ineffective communication, which can be verbal or non-verbal.

Enjoyment in practice is not about how many people you see it is about how many people you can connect with. Be yourself and not the person you think you should or others think you should be. That leads to self-doubt and burnout. Help people associate their care with being able to achieve or be able to do what is important to them. Then you can help them to effect change. Join people on their journey rather than pushing them to where you think they want to go. You will be in your flow and then find people will want care, rather than having to be told they need it.

Do what you love.

Wisdom #29

Martin Harvey BSc, MChiro, DC

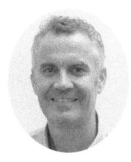

Martin is inspired by the potential that chiropractic care has to transform the health of our communities. He is the immediate past President of the Australian Spinal Research Foundation, is a sought-after speaker and leads a multi-doctor family practice in Melbourne. He teaches chiropractors around the world how to better communicate their value.

Martin was awarded the Chiropractors Association of Australia (Vic) Chiropractor of the Year Award for 2012, Parker Seminars 2010 International Chiropractor of the Year and was honoured as an inaugural Member of the Australasian College of Chiropractors.

Wisdom from a reformed chirovangelist.

Undoubtedly the most important lesson I have learned as a chiropractor, I learned from being a chirovangelist. What was the lesson (and what's a chirovangelist?) I hear you ask?

What is a chirovangelist?

Have you ever had this happen to you? You're in some sort of social setting, a party, or out at dinner and someone asks you what you do. You say you're a chiropractor and the person's response has been, "Wow, you must give a great massage", or "So you're a back-cracker", or "Thank God I've never needed a chiropractor", or "So I guess chiropractory is getting more accepted these days?"

Or have you ever had someone who has had care, say something like, "I don't need to come anymore because I feel better", or "I went to a chiropractor and they just want you to come back again and again so they can get more money", or "My doctor told me I shouldn't have chiropractic because I have osteoporosis".

Doesn't it grate? Doesn't it piss you off?

In my observation there are 2 common ways that we chiropractors respond. The first is the chirowimp. This is where we don't want to make a scene, or we feel a bit tired or a bit rushed, or we don't want the confrontation so we just let it go. It goes like this. They say "Thank God I've never needed a chiropractor" and we say, "Uh, yes, lucky you". They say, "I feel better so I don't need to go back" and we say, "Oh, okay".

Meanwhile on the inside we're making all sorts of rationalisations. "Well, I don't want to seem pushy", or "Chiropractic's not for everyone" or "People that stupid don't deserve Chiropractic". Then later on, as you think about it, you kick yourself because you know that you are letting them hang on to their misperception and, in some way, robbing them of the chance to understand a bigger perspective on health.

I have a confession to make – I've been a chirowimp. And the reality is that, as well as not helping people see a different view of health, you feel the deep, dark pain of regret.

The second way we respond is as a chirovangelist. This is where we really want them to get a different perspective. So we give it to them. With both barrels. The core beliefs of the chirovangelist are that to get more people to have chiropractic care we need to just "tell the story" and that if they knew what we knew, they would do what we do.

It goes something like this. They say "Thank God I've never needed a chiropractor", and we say, "You know what? That's not what chiropractic is about at all! If you want to be as healthy as possible, and develop to your full potential, you simply cannot do it unless your nervous system is free of interference."

As a chirovangelist we use this blunt approach at all times, including in the practice. They say, "I don't need to come in anymore because I feel great" and our response is, "Well you can't tell whether you're healthy by how you feel. Don't you know that subluxations are serious! Would you wait until you had a rotten tooth to see the dentist? Would you wait until your car broke down before you got it serviced? Well, your spine is your lifeline, so why not look after that too?" And on the inside we feel like you have really shown them. I have another confession to make. I've been a chirovangelist too.

And being a chirovangelist works. A little bit. I had some people who I spoke to at parties who decided to have chiropractic care. But most didn't. I had a lot of people change the topic, walk off or just nod along until I stopped ranting. There were some people who experienced my super-direct chirovangelist approach in the office and it seemed to result in them continuing care. But most just hung around for another visit or 2, then disappeared.

And to some of them I must have looked like a presumptive arsehole. Because I tried to make them wrong to think the way they did. You see, people say those things, not to annoy you, but because that is what they believe. They have a different world-view of health.

The chiropractic paradigm says that your body is meant to

be healthy. It's designed to be self-healing, self-regulating and self-developing. That chiropractic harnesses the power of the master control system, your nervous system, to help your whole body work better, and when your body works better your whole life (and future) is better.

Is this the common view of health in our communities? No. Most people view health as being about how you feel. If you feel good you're healthy, feel bad and you're sick. Most people believe that their bodies are weak and vulnerable, and whether they get sick or not is due to genes, germs and just bad luck. They see Chiropractic as a slightly alternative, possibly dangerous way of treating uncomplicated back pain.

Is it any wonder that they will believe and say things that don't fit our paradigm?

So I was a chirovangelist for the first few years of practice. I would psyche myself up to "tell the story" and fight for what I knew people needed to know. I was a chirovangelist until I realised that telling people doesn't work. So why is it that being a chirovangelist and telling the story doesn't work? Why doesn't sharing the truth set them free?

It's because when we are being chirovangelists we are selling our beliefs without any regard for theirs. It's a bit like if you asked someone out for a date, then when you picked them up you whipped out a condom and said "how about it?" It's all about your beliefs and what you want and nothing about them and what's important to them.

Even more than this, we make them wrong for what they believe. We are strongly wired to dread (and avoid) being wrong. While academically we all know that we can't be right all the time, we still hate it when we are made wrong for a belief we hold. In psychology literature they talk about being made wrong as reducing our sense of self-efficacy, our ability to look after ourselves in the world. This, at some level feels unsafe, and so we have a strong emotional drive to feel "right", which feels safe.

When we make people wrong in their health choices or understanding of chiropractic, the best possible outcome is that they ignore us. The worst one is that we evoke confirmation bias and they go looking for all the reasons they were right and we were wrong, which then reinforces their existing beliefs! We "tell the story", trying to win them over to a chiropractic view of the world and inadvertently reinforce their existing beliefs. So the first part of the lesson is that we have to stop being a chirovangelist and stop telling the story!

So, what do we do instead?

Fortunately, chiropractors are not the only people trying to change people's behavior. There is an entire field (the influence literature) that researches why people do what they do, and what we can do to ethically influence them to adopt healthier behaviours. The influence literature includes research from psychology, neuroscience, behavioural economics and marketing and has some huge lessons for how we can craft our communication in a way that gives our beautiful chiropractic message in a way that matters. To them. Chiropractic has a huge advantage because everyone has things that they have to do, love to do and see as their identity to do. These are the things that give their life meaning. Whether it's being a super-mum, a CEO or a golfer, everyone has what I describe as their lifestyle values. And there is no lifestyle value that isn't improved by having a body that works better. Once people realise that Chiropractic helps them be better at the things they love to do and see as their identity to do, the time, energy and money they spend on having chiropractic care stops being a cost and starts being an investment. We are all looking to reduce costs but never looking to reduce investments.

To get to this, the first lesson is to start by agreeing with them. I know it's counter-intuitive to agree when someone says that "Chiropractic is dangerous" or "You're a back cracker", or "I don't need to come in because I feel good"!

One of the most powerful strategies from the influence literature to do this is one called, "Yes.. and". It comes from the world of improv theatre (it's one of the fundamental rules of improv). It's an amazing way of avoiding making people with different health beliefs wrong when you communicate about chiropractic because step 1 is "yes", where you agree with them.

Not that they are right necessarily but their belief is reasonable. "I can see why you might think that Chiropractic is dangerous", "I have heard other people describe us as back-crackers", "I understand why you would want to stop care now that you are feeling better".

The paradox of using "Yes.. and" is that as soon as you agree with them, they are immediately more interested in what you say next, which is the "... and" part. This is where you get to tell the chiropractic story, just in a way that is relevant to them! "... and another perspective is that Chiropractic has one of the best safety records in healthcare" or, "... and the crack sound is a sign that there has been a change in pressure in the joints of the spine as the spine has been gently and specifically adjusted" or "... and another view is that continuing care is likely to help you minimise the chance of a relapse."

A key distinction in using "Yes... and" is that it is not "Yes... but". The power in the strategy is in agreeing with them and "but" negates that agreement. So the lesson is that we need to stop telling the story. We need to avoid being both a chirowimp and a chirovangelist and become a chiroinfluencer. Step 1 is to agree that it is understandable that they believe what they believe, because once we are on the same page we can lead them to an understanding of how, quite simply, life goes better with Chiropractic.

Vismai Schonfelder DC, Marty Cook DC

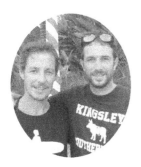

Vismai graduated from RMIT in Melbourne in 1998 with a keen interest in family chiropractic care. He has authored 2 books which he uses as practice building tools and he coaches via his online platform My Chiropractic Sweet Spot, focused on assisting chiropractors searching for life coherence. Vismai speaks regularly at seminars worldwide.

He is married to Jyoti with two teenage children Dali and Finn and the family love to travel and experience new cultures. In 2011 they began volunteering in India with other chiropractors, and have donated around 8 million days of school as a result.

A 2006 graduate from RMIT, Marty practiced in Melbourne where he held a board member position on the CAA (Vic) branch. In 2008, he decided to move to the UK before finally settling permanently in The Netherlands, where he purchased the practice he was working in.

Marty has a passion for SOT, developmental functional neurology and helping children, leading him to a board position on SOTO Europe and completing his Masters in Paediatrics in 2019. He enjoys communicating the importance of developing a culture within practice which supports the growth and development of associates, creating successful associate driven practices.

Long Term Friendship and Chiropractic Business.

Associates won't build your practice. They never have, they aren't currently, and they never will. Principal chiropractors frequently hire associates envisioning practice growth with all the perceived benefits, yet are left with financial stress, a resentful associate and practice instability. The opposite of their dream practice. The finger of blame gets pointed at everyone involved, resulting in even more instability, which is eventually felt by patients.

Yet, thriving associate-driven practices do exist. So what is it that separates the successful associate-driven practices from the unsuccessful?

When I was a recent graduate, this question was constantly on my mind. How could I find a position where I was happy, successful and fulfilled, while avoiding a position that would result in me becoming another "failed associate" statistic? What was it that I was supposed to be looking for? While at the time I couldn't label it, my experience over the coming years would assist me in identifying it as "culture".

The culture of a practice forms a key element to its stability and growth. The culture of a practice describes the ideals and customs that guide decision making, direction and belief system of the practice. Having a clearly established culture for employing associates, nurturing their development and providing ongoing support throughout their employment, are the foundations that provide a pathway to success for both associate and principal chiropractor. Furthermore, this provides an opportunity for the development of long-term friendship in chiropractic business. This is surprisingly rare in chiropractic. It shouldn't be.

Employing an associate is an important step for the growth of a chiropractic business. However, it is essential to have an associate-focused culture already developed prior to employing someone. The absence of an existing well-engineered culture will result in errors being made, expectations not being met and friction between employee and employer. This is where most chiropractic practices fail when trying to grow.

Of all the aspects that contribute to the creation of long-term friendship and chiropractic business, communication is perhaps the most important. While overlooked by many chiropractors, creating an open space for discussion provides both the chiropractor and associate with the opportunity to connect. Frequent and structured communication can mitigate problems early on. Every Monday, I would meet with Vismai for lunch to discuss issues that had presented themselves in practice. Chiropractic technique questions, ideas for better communication and thoughts surrounding philosophy, were all regularly discussed.

Sometimes lunch was busy with discussion, sometimes it was quieter with thought and reflection. These periods contributed to us both understanding and growing together. This time together was extended into regularly spending time together with his family at their home, attending seminars and even going on holidays together.

Part of an associate-focused culture is providing the

associate with security, which takes many forms. When commencing work with Vismai, I was provided with a large patient base. As an associate, having a patient base to walk into, or having a long list of new patients waiting for appointments provides stability financially. More importantly, it is one of the first steps to the establishment of trust between associate and principal chiropractor. Knowing that Vismai had the skills to build a practice to the point where he required more chiropractors to meet demand, gave me confidence in Vismai as a great chiropractor, communicator and leader.

The flip side is also true. The practice owner should anticipate and even demand regular contact outside of the office because this helps to nip small problems in the bud before they develop into larger ones. A rhythm to these meetings is a helpful structure and provides a reliable platform for deepening the relationship.

As a practice owner, you have a social responsibility to be a skilful business operator. You can't "have your cake and eat it" by reaping in all the rewards but not facing responsibility on new patient flow, retention techniques and a well-rounded, bulletproof office culture. We invited the next associate into our business only after they had passed our 3-step, 3-month-long interview process and only if they either walked into an existing patient base or a new patient waiting list of at least 50 people.

Of course, developing a great business takes time. The most important component of implementation is not actually the speed at which you create your stable and thriving business, but more importantly the sequential order in which it is done.

We built our successful, turn-key, associate-driven practice using 3 main phases - in this sequence too. Our office was so stable that we took a year-long sabbatical, had only 2 phone calls from the office that year and returned to 10% growth.

Phase 1 Foundations:
· The entrepreneur chiropractor mindset.
· Understanding chiropractic business//private life coherence
· The anatomy of my chiropractic business.
· Financing my life as a chiropractor.

Phase 2 Going vertical: Understanding the values of people who love you.
· Creating your total sales package by ultra-targeting the people who love you.
· The associate interview process.
· Maintaining your associate chiropractors.

Phase 3 Going horizontal: Scaling your business and positioning your practice more broadly in your community.

   Get this sequence correct and you can do really well as the owner and associate. And who knows, you might end up making great friends for life - and that is a worthy pursuit.

Wisdom #30

Tony Croke BAppSci (Chiro) DC

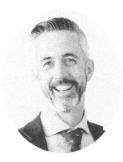 *RMIT graduate Tony has studied deeply what it takes to earn the right to be called somebody's chiropractor. It's an honour he doesn't take lightly. He has served the profession in a number of roles since 1992 including as a founding member of the board of the SCCT.*

Named 2010 Chiropractor of the Year for the Australian state of Victoria for his work in protecting access to chiropractic care for Australian children, Tony himself is a proud father of 3. Of his children, 2 have gone on to become chiropractors. When he's out of the office, Tony describes himself as an unskilled but enthusiastic surfer and snow-skier.

The power of listening

I'd been in practice more than 20 years. I'd spoken at chiropractic seminars locally and internationally. I had a brilliant, beautiful wife and 3 amazing children. I'd been recognised as Chiropractor of the Year by my state association and lauded for my work in promoting and protecting the chiropractic profession. Together with my wife, Tiff, I'd grown a busy practice in a wonderful community.

Yet, here I was, sitting at my desk, alone, looking out of the window into the garden of our beautiful home, contemplating a thought I'd never had before.

Maybe my family would be better without me?

Practice had stagnated, referrals and profits had dried up. My relationships with my wife and children were in various states of disrepair. I felt tired, deflated and guilty that I wasn't bringing joy to those around me. Especially Tiff, who had supported and helped grow our practice and our family. I felt like I was letting her down and I felt that I was letting Chiropractic down by not being able to get the message out to my community in a way that made them bang down the doors trying to get their spines checked!

Perhaps if I was out of the way, Tiff could run our practice better without me in it, my children would be happier and the world would be a better place.

It's awful to think back on that time and realise how far down a dark path my mind had wandered.

Thankfully, the realisation that my thinking had become so self-destructive was enough of a jolt to get me contemplating and creating change.

Tiff is a counsellor and has amazing insight gained from years of training and practice, combined with a dogged determination to learn from her circumstances and past missteps. Me, not so much.

She and I would often talk about the dynamics of families, relationships and communication. Some of our conversations sunk in, but some I let slide by; especially if it felt a little close to the bone.

I'd grown up in a benevolent dictatorship of do-what-you're-told parenting. It was OK most of the time, but didn't really stand up to the pressure of difficult conversations in tough circumstances. If I'm honest, I'd grown my practice in a similarly authoritarian way; caring and with my clients' best interests at heart, but in the end, it was "my way or the highway". Despite my best efforts, I often defaulted back to that approach in my parenting too.

In the early years, I watched my practice grow through enthusiastically telling the chiropractic story, unaware that aspects of my communication style were sowing the seeds of future frustration, both in practice and at home.

When power is the instrument of influence, it only continues to work if the power balance stays in one's favor. As my children grew, that balance shifted. And as my community was given an almost infinite number of health information sources with the growth of the internet, and a local proliferation of health practitioners of various types, trainers, Pilates and yoga studios, my level of influence in my community decreased too.

Neither my children nor my practice members were going to put up with "Because I said so …" as an answer to their questions any more. In fact, that had stopped working a while ago, I was just catching up with the facts.

Sitting there at my desk, I realised that my communication style was the "subluxation" in my life.

So, I went back to the foundations of chiropractic philosophy which have served me so well in the past. It was there that I found something so obvious, but so fundamentally vital that it has profoundly influenced me ever since.

The Normal Complete Cycle, also known in Chiropractic as the "safety pin cycle", depicts the 2-way communication between brain cell and tissue cell via the nervous system's motor and sensory pathways.

In my early understanding of Chiropractic, I focused on

the idea of the reduction of subluxation improving normal outflow of mental impulses from the brain to the body. As my understanding of the neurological impact of the chiropractic adjustment has grown over the years, I have learned that the normalization of feedback from the body to the brain is at least as important as the reduction of interference to motor signals.

In a sense, I pondered, a chiropractic adjustment helps our body listen to itself more effectively. And in that moment, I realised that was not just a neurophysiological requirement for health. It was the solution to my current collection of problems.

Of course, Tiff had been gently trying to tell me this for years. But was I ready to listen? Not likely! However, the cumulative effects of my choices were now painful enough that change was the only option.

I knew I didn't have the skills or knowledge to get out of this situation on my own.

I started working with a chiropractor friend to radically change the approach in our practice communication at every level. We agreed to a set of 3 key words against which everything we did would be measured. From here on, we aimed to be "remarkable, enlivening and loving".

We asked the team to be brave enough to let us know if they saw anyone - including me - doing our jobs in less than a remarkable, enlivening and loving way. Despite my hard-wired defensiveness, they cared enough about the people we served to persist with this approach. The more I received their feedback as an exciting opportunity to improve (rather than a personal insult!), the more our relationships with our clients and within our team grew.

I worked with Tiff to forge those links between honesty,

accountability and success in our practice culture. Even more importantly, I stumbled and fumbled my way towards implementing those same changes in my family life... and continue to do so.

So, what does it mean to listen?

First, let's talk about what it's not. It's not giving advice or making suggestions. It's not disagreeing, judging or blaming. It's not reassuring, consoling or trying to make a person think positive; and it's definitely not waiting for someone to stop talking so that you can explain your opinion about their experience.

Listening involves being with a person where they are, and feeling what they might be feeling. It's feeding back to them the content of what they've said, along with how you think that might make them feel. And don't worry if you get it wrong, people will appreciate you making the effort and help you get it right if you're a little off-track.

Listening is letting your eyes well up when a wife tells you about what it's like to have her husband go into assisted living and being apart from him for the first time in 65 years.

It's truly acknowledging and sitting with the fear of a single mum who needs to be able to work to provide for her family but has a painful lower back injury.

It's being defenseless in the face of a new client who had a bad experience with their previous chiropractor and, out of desperation, is giving Chiropractic one more shot.

Listening opens doors and breaks down barriers. It heals hearts and calms minds.

When we seek to understand what matters to the people we work with before we offer them any kind of solution, we create a space where they can hear themselves think. Once that happens, then we can explain how Chiropractic might help them get what they want.

And more importantly, we've created a relationship that bonds us together and builds trust. When we do that over and over, we build a life of rich connections in every part of our lives.

As I write this in June 2020, we are deep in the Covid-19 pandemic. Unlike some jurisdictions, in Australia we have been able to stay open to serve our community. In the most challenging time in most people's living memory, our practice has grown by over 30%.

I credit Tiff, my team and the work we've all done to build those deep connections with people so that we are seen as a safe and trusted space in the most difficult of times.

That's the power of listening.

Resources:

If you're looking for somewhere to start to learn more about listening, these are the best two books I've ever read on the subject. But neither of them will teach you as much as your family and your practice members can.

Covey, S. (1989). *The 7 habits of highly effective people.* New York, Simon and Schuster.

Gordon, T. (1970). *PET: Parent effectiveness training: the tested new way to raise responsible children.* PH Wyden.

Jorge Compos BSc, DC

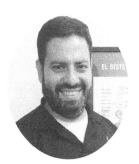

Jorge Campos DC earned a BSc degree from Texas A&M University, is a 2009 graduate of Palmer College of Chiropractic in Davenport, Iowa and is a member of the Academy of Chiropractic Philosophers.

In 2019, after 10 years of private practice, he moved from Chile to join the Sherman College staff as the director of the Reach Out And Recruit Department (ROAR). Dr Campos has helped with the exponential growth of the chiropractic profession in South America, and he is passionate about bringing Chiropractic to the world.

Blood, sweat, and tears: my path to becoming a chiropractor.

I will never forget that winter afternoon in June 1999, in Santiago, Chile. On that day, my life would change forever. That would be the first time my ears heard about the science, art, and philosophy of Chiropractic from the mouth of Dr H Lee Eller. Dr Eller was a chiropractor who was visiting my country with his wife Faye, because his son Stephen had just finished a Christian mission in southern Chile.

During his time in Chile, Stephen and I became good friends, and we still are to this day. I was born and raised in the city of Santiago, and for that reason I offered myself as a tour guide to Stephen and his parents. During that tour day, Dr Eller told me about the purpose of Chiropractic. He explained to me how Chiropractic had an impact on the nervous system, health, and life in general.

That same day, Dr Eller asked me what I wanted to do with my life. I replied that I really liked the human body and biology, but that I could not imagine myself prescribing medications or doing surgeries on people.

Therefore, the closest thing to my interest that I could study in Chile was physical therapy. Due to my new fascination with Chiropractic and all the questions I asked Dr Eller, he asked me if I would like to study Chiropractic. I replied, "yes" with a sad voice, because unfortunately the chiropractic career did not exist in Chile, therefore it would be impossible for me to study it.

I knew that it was very expensive to study in the US and I was from a very humble family, so a US education was not within my reach. In fact, I was the first person in my family who wanted to pursue a college education. I wanted to break the cycle of poverty in my life, and I wanted to do it through professional education.

Dr Eller listened to my answer and just stared at me thoughtfully as we continued on the tour. At the end of the day, Dr Eller looked at me seriously and said, "If you really want to be a chiropractor, I am going to make you a proposal. I will let you come and live in my house in California. My wife and I will give you a roof and food, but the cost of your education will depend on you."

When I heard those words, I knew that Dr Eller had realised how my energy decreased during the tour. I was saddened because I had discovered such a wonderful career and I would not be able to study it in Chile.

His extremely generous invitation took me by surprise. At the time, I had no idea how I was going to pay for an education in the US. Due to all of my doubts, I told Dr Eller, "I am going to think about his proposal. Thank you very much for this wonderful offer."

I knew that neither my family nor I had the resources to pay for a college education in the US, but at the same time, I was fascinated with this new discovery in my life called Chiropractic. Although I was just a 21-year-old boy, I knew I should try to become a chiropractor. If I tried and failed, at least my conscience would be at peace that I had made the effort. If I did not take that risk, then it would become a regret that would haunt me for the rest of my life.

So, at the age of 21, I made the decision to live a life without regrets and that I would go and seek my fortune in the United States.

Once I had made this decision, I called Dr Eller and said with great conviction, "I will. I am going to study Chiropractic". I will never forget the warmth I felt in my chest when I said those words. I could feel this new passion burning inside of me. That year I did not go to college in Chile to study physical therapy, I worked for the Marriott hotel in Santiago for 12 months instead, to save money.

I still remember the nervousness of coming to the United States with only U$3,000 in my pocket, that I had saved working for the Marriott.

I did not know how I was going to achieve my education, but I did know that I had already made an unwavering commitment to do it.

I started my college course at Butte College, California. That year I paid the international student fee of US $2,000 per semester (a high fee compared to the US$250 that California residents paid).

After paying for my first semester, I only had a U$1,000 left in my pocket, so I looked for a job at the college and worked as many hours as possible to collect the other thousand that I needed for the following semester. The second semester came, I paid for it, and I continued studying and working hard.

When the third semester came, I only had U$1,000 in my pocket and I needed an extra thousand to pay for my student fees. During that time, I had been a very hardworking student, I had excellent grades, and belonged to an honour student society called Phi Theta Kappa. Because of that, Butte College gave me a special scholarship and downgraded my payments to residency tuition. In this way, I was able to continue my education at this community college and also save money for chiropractic school.

When the time came to pursue my Bachelor's Degree, I did not have enough money to pay for college, so I went to the library, ordered a book containing 5,000 scholarships, and read each scholarship requirement, one by one.

In the book, 4,998 scholarships required being a citizen or resident of the United States to apply. It was scary that my future depended on just 2 scholarships that I could apply for.

I filled out the applications and I asked God to help me fulfil my dream of becoming a chiropractor.

I was so joyful and grateful when I received a letter from the Texas A&M University-Commerce saying that I was awarded the Phi Theta Kappa scholarship. My prayers had been heard and the hope of becoming a chiropractor was still alive. I continued to work very hard, and after completing my Bachelors, I was accepted by Palmer College of Chiropractic in Davenport, Iowa.

I was finally just steps away from achieving my goal and

dream of studying Chiropractic. My first semester was very hard. Not only because I was studying many science courses, but I was also working to survive. I started Palmer as an international student and I did not have access to student loans. However, it was a real blessing that my Green Card was approved that year.

Because of that, I was able to apply for student loans, and finally able to focus 100% on studying Chiropractic. However, there is something you do not know, something very intimate that I want to share with you. In order to pay for Palmer's first semester, I had to make the decision not to see my family for 4 years. If I bought a plane ticket, I would have had to spend over £1,000 dollars, which was the money I was saving to go to chiropractic college.

I also worked hard in fast food joints, in construction, and cleaning the John Deere factory at night. In addition to that, I often sold my blood at plasma centres. They paid me US$30 for half a litre, which was money that my wife and I needed so we could eat. There is a well-known saying that goes, "That cost me blood, sweat, and tears". In my case, that saying was a reality. To become a chiropractor I sold my blood, I sweated working very hard in construction and cleaning, and I cried many times because I could not see my family for 4 years.

The question then is, was it worth it? My answer is a categorical YES.

Being able to return to Chile in 2009 to be the only chiropractor for more than 300,000 people was an unforgettable experience. Travelling around Chile doing television and radio interviews and telling the chiropractic story to people, was an honour for me. There are hundreds of stories that I could share with you about my experience as a chiropractor in Chile.

However, I just want to focus on one very special story that I want to share with you.

During one of my radio interviews, a medical doctor called, very upset, asking why a non-medical quack was talking about the nervous system and its effect on people's health. The interview was a little tense after that call, but I continued to tell the story of chiropractic. I did it in a firm, fearless, and very secure way.

About a month after that interview, a patient who was a man of very few words, got up from my chiropractic table, and with tears in his eyes said to me, "Thank you doctor for saving my life." This man already had two spinal surgeries without success, and he suffered from sciatic pain in both legs. I smiled at him and I said, "I am very happy that you feel better about your pain, but I did not save your life."

After saying those words, I saw his wife crying next to him, which really caught my attention. This man looked at me again and said, "No doctor, you saved my life. I was in my room with a gun in my hand thinking of taking my own life. However, my wife knocked on my door and invited me to listen to the radio. I listened to you speak with so such passion and conviction that I decided to try one last time to improve my health with this new unfamiliar thing called Chiropractic. If I had not listened to you on the radio, I would have already taken my own life."

I teared up, gave him a big hug, and thanked him for telling me that story. That day, I discovered that Chiropractic goes far beyond removing pain or improving mobility. Chiropractic exists to improve the quality of life for every individual on this planet. Now I know that Chiropractic improves, optimises, and saves lives.

From that experience, and many more, I know without any doubt that all those sacrifices that I made to become a chiropractor were absolutely worth it, and I would do it all over again.

Wisdom #31

James Chestnut MSc, DC, CCWP

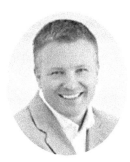 *James L Chestnut has been studying human wellness and prevention for over 30 years. He holds a Bachelor of Physical Education degree, a Master of Science degree in exercise physiology with a specialisation in neuromuscular adaptation, is a Doctor of Chiropractic and has a post-graduate certification in Wellness Lifestyle. Dr Chestnut is also the author of Live Right for Your Species Type.*

In 2009 Dr Chestnut was awarded the Parker Seminars Chiropractor of the Year award and in 2007 he won the International Chiropractors Association Chiropractic Educator of the Year Award. The Wellness Lifestyle Certification Program he developed has set the standard for evidence-based lifestyle intervention, based on the human genetic requirements regarding nutrition, exercise, and energy expenditure, belief systems, thoughts and emotions and social interaction.

Evidence of Bias Against SMT/Adjustment in the Peer-Reviewed Literature

When it comes to clinical evidence regarding the benefits of chiropractic SMT/adjustment, there can be no argument that, by far, the vast majority of available research evidence is focused on non-specific spinal (in particular low back) pain, disability, and pain and disability-related quality of life. Whether you agree with this research or clinical focus or not, the irrefutable truth is that non-specific low back pain, and other non-specific spinal health and quality of life issues, represent a pandemic health crisis and a healthcare financial crisis, with a huge proportion of patients seeking chiropractic care, and, based on the currently available research evidence, is the only area where chiropractors can currently make evidence-based claims of superior clinical benefit.

I am not suggesting that there is evidence that reduced pain and disability and improved spine-related quality of life are the only benefits elicited from chiropractic SMT/adjustment, I am factually stating that these are currently the only benefits that can be validly classified as evidence-based. There are other benefits that, based on less than conclusive clinical evidence, basic science evidence, and/or clinical experience, can validly be classified as evidence-informed, but that is not the topic of this discussion. I have always highly encouraged, and have donated ample time and money to, more research into the global effects/benefits of regular chiropractic adjustment/SMT care. The facts are that such research is lacking, has been for decades, and that this has not been amply addressed. The onus is not on those who ask for evidence regarding claims of benefit, the onus is on those who make claims of benefit. This is both fair and ethical. We need to fund, conduct, and publish valid research! That said, this discussion is about the level of evidence for chiropractic SMT/adjustment for non-specific spinal health issues.

There are millions and millions of people suffering from such spinal health issues and these people need and deserve to have access to the most evidence-based care. For decades I have been making the evidence-based argument that chiropractic

SMT/adjustment (and general spinal and overall fitness exercises and healthy lifestyle advice) represents the most evidence-based first care option in terms of effectiveness, cost-effectiveness, and safety.

I contend that, based on a fair interpretation of the peer-reviewed clinical evidence, of all the possible interventions for non-cancerous, non-infectious, non-traumatic instability neuromusculospinal health issues (uncomplicated or non-specific spinal health issues), the most evidence-based with respect to effectiveness, cost-effectiveness, and safety, is chiropractic thrust SMT/adjustment (and general spinal and overall fitness exercises and healthy lifestyle advice). This is true for interventions within and outside chiropractic education and scope of practice.

I realise that this is not always the conclusion of systematic reviews and/or clinical guidelines, which often rate the evidence for SMT as similar, or inferior to, other interventions. I contend that this is due to a bias against SMT in clinical studies, in systematic reviews, and in the evidence rating scales such as the JADAD scale, due to a failure to take into account variables which can significantly affect outcomes such as dose of care, timing of outcome measures in relation to end of active care, and differentiation between thrust SMT and non-thrust mobilisations.

Most clinicians simply rely on the conclusions of systematic reviews, as they lack the familiarity with the literature, scientific methodological expertise, and/or time to properly critique such reviews by reading each individual study reviewed, assess its methodological validity, and/or recognise which studies have been excluded, based on selection criteria. Most clinicians are also unaware that the JADAD and other study quality rating scales do not differentiate between studies that include 2 or 3 SMT sessions vs studies that include 8-12 SMT sessions; studies that measure outcomes weeks or months after the last SMT session vs immediately after the last SMT session; or studies that include only non-thrust mobilisations vs thrust SMT.

As Bronfort et al. pointed out in their 2008 review in *The Spine Journal* regarding the lack of standardisation of dose of care and timing of collecting outcome measures data in the published studies, "The number of SMT treatments varied from 1 to 24 and follow-up from immediate posttreatment to 3 years."[12] Inexplicably, and pathetically, little has changed since 2008; the lack of standardisation in SMT study methodology makes lumping all these studies together into a single systematic review invalid and using the JADAD scale or any other study quality rating scale cannot correct for this issue.

This lack of standardisation of dose of care and follow-up time also creates large heterogeneity of results which is used to justify downgrading the level of evidence for SMT in systematic reviews. As an example, from the recent 2017 Paige et al. systematic review in JAMA, "The quality of evidence was judged as moderate that treatment with SMT was associated with improved pain and function in patients with acute low back pain, which was downgraded from high, due to inconsistency of results."[13]

In other words, the actual data analysis showed high quality

---

12 Bronfort et al. Evidence-informed management of chronic low back pain with spinal manipulation and mobilisation. The Spine Journal 2008 (8): 213-225.
13 Paige et al. (2017) Association of Spinal Manipulative Therapy with Clinical Benefit and Harm for Acute Low Back Pain. Systematic Review and Meta-analysis. JAMA;317(14):1451-1460

evidence that SMT was associated with improved pain and function, which by the way would make SMT the clear leader in quality of evidence, but the authors chose to downgrade the level of evidence to moderate because of heterogeneity (inconsistency) of results. The most frustrating part is that the authors make no effort to explain this heterogeneity of results based on dose of care, timing of outcome measurement, or thrust vs non-thrust SMT interventions.

As a point of example, the highest rated study in terms of quality in the Paige et al. review is the Hancock et al. study published in the Lancet that concluded that SMT failed to provide any clinically relevant benefit in terms of time to recovery, pain, or disability. This Hancock et al. study is consistently rated as the highest quality study of SMT in systematic reviews. There is no better example of the shortcomings of the JADAD study quality rating scale. The Hancock study receives a score of 8 out of 10 (very high) NOT because it is well designed to answer the questions it poses or that its overall methodological design or conclusions lack evidence of bias, but because it was well-blinded and thus lacks bias in terms of data collection and analysis, which is the most highly weighted aspect of the JADAD rating system.

The methodological problems of this study, and the bias of the authors, is clear to see for anyone who understands research methodology and is willing to read the full study rather than just the abstract. Firstly, every patient in the study receives paracetamol 4 times a day, including the so-called non-treatment group as well as the NSAID and SMT groups. This is like assessing the effectiveness of paracetamol in a study where every subject receives SMT; it is methodologically absurd. If you want to compare SMT to paracetamol, or SMT to the NSAID diclofenac, or if you want to compare diclofenac to paracetamol, then you do so by having groups that receive one treatment or the other, as well as groups who receive placebo, and then compare outcomes.

Secondly, the SMT group did not receive SMT, they received mobilisations which were labelled as SMT. "Participants allocated to spinal manipulative therapy had treatment 2 or 3 times per week [at the physiotherapist's discretion] to a maximum of 12 treatments over 4 weeks [the average was 2.3 treatments per week]." "Most participants had several low-velocity mobilisation techniques [232/239, 97%] with a small proportion also having high-velocity thrust techniques [12/239, 5%]."[14]

Only 5% of the SMT group received thrust SMT, the other 95% received mobilisations. Most disturbing is that the authors falsely claim that thrust SMT and mobilisations are clinically synonymous and use a bogus citation to support their unfounded claim. "A systematic review of spinal manipulation concluded that there is no evidence that high-velocity spinal manipulation is more effective than low-velocity spinal mobilisation, or that the profession of the manipulator affects the effectiveness of treatment."[14]

The reference they provide is not a systematic review of spinal manipulation at all and certainly not a systematic review of a comparison of thrust spinal manipulation vs mobilisations or the effects of the profession of the manipulator on outcomes. The study they cite is a review of NSAIDs: van Tulder MW, Scholten RJ, Koes BW, Deyo RA. Nonsteroidal anti-inflammatory drugs

14 Hancock, M.J. et al. (2007) Assessment of diclofenac [Voltaren] or spinal manipulative therapy, or both, in addition to recommended first-line treatment for acute low back pain: a randomised controlled trial. Lancet. 2007;370:1638-1643

for low back pain: a systematic review within the framework of the Cochrane Collaboration Back Review Group. *Spine 2000;* **25:** 2501–13.

Here is what the authors conclude. "If patients have high rates of recovery with baseline care [paracetamol] and no clinically worthwhile benefit from the addition of diclofenac or spinal manipulative therapy, then GPs can manage patients confidently without exposing them to increased risks and costs associated with NSAIDs or spinal manipulative therapy."[14]

The authors cite no evidence of increased risk or costs associated with SMT compared to paracetamol, and they also fail to provide a shred of evidence of "high rates of recovery with baseline [paracetamol] care". This is understandable; there has never been a shred of evidence for the effectiveness of paracetamol, despite the fact that it was considered the gold standard first-line medical care option in virtually every medical clinical guideline for low back pain treatment. One wonders how GPs "can manage patients confidently" with an intervention that has zero evidence of effectiveness, and ample evidence of ineffectiveness. I guess they can at least feel confident knowing they are not exposing patients to the increased risk and costs of dangerous and ineffective SMT! Give me a break, the bias against SMT, and for an intervention with not a shred of evidence, is pathetically obvious, intellectually dishonest, and scientifically unfounded. Keep in mind, this study not only passed peer-review, it is consistently rated as one of the highest quality studies of SMT in systematic reviews and has been extensively used to downgrade the level of evidence for SMT.

Contrast this with the systematic review by Hidalgo et al. published in the *Journal of Manual and Manipulative Therapy.*

This is the only systematic review that I am aware of that distinguishes between thrust vs non-thrust SMT. "Two stages of LBP were categorised; combined acute-subacute and chronic. Further sub-classification was made according to MT intervention: MT1 (manipulation); MT2 (mobilisation and soft-tissue-techniques); and MT3 (MT1 combined with MT2).[15]

The authors conclude that thrust manipulation (MT1) is superior to non-thrust manipulation or mobilisations (MT2) and to placebo for both acute-subacute and chronic low back pain. "Firstly, in comparison to previous reports of limited evidence showing no difference between true and sham manipulation, the results of this systematic review show moderate to strong evidence for the beneficial effects of [thrust] manipulation in comparison to sham manipulation." "These differences are demonstrated in terms of pain relief, functional improvement, and overall-health and quality of life improvements in the short-term for all stages of LBP."[15] This rating makes thrust SMT the most highly rated intervention for both acute-subacute and chronic low back pain. Imagine if they also controlled for valid doses of care.

It's not just that many SMT studies do not include manipulation, many also include only 1-3 SMT treatments. The results of these studies then get pooled in systematic reviews with the very few studies that include valid doses of thrust SMT care. What do you think this does to the rating of the level of evidence of effectiveness for SMT in systematic reviews? I remind you again, neither dose of care nor timing of outcome measures, nor thrust vs non-thrust SMT is accounted for by the

---

15 Fritz, J.M. et al. (2015) Early physical therapy vs usual care in patients with recent-onset low back pain: A randomised clinical trial. JAMA 314 (14): 1459-1467.

JADAD quality rating scale.

For just a few of many examples. A study published in the Spine Journal in 2016 that concluded that SMT elicited no clinically meaningful benefit for patients with chronic low back pain only included 3 once-weekly sessions of SMT over a month, and the outcomes were assessed a full month after cessation of care.[16] Another study in 2015 published in JAMA included 3-4 sessions of SMT over 4 weeks, measured outcomes at 3 months and 1 year, and concluded SMT elicited no clinically meaningful benefit.[17]

Not only are 2-3 SMT treatments not representative of clinical practice, this dose of care is not reflective of the evidence found in the peer-reviewed literature. As Haas et al. point out in one of the few valid studies conducted on dose of care, "Therefore 12 sessions of SMT is the current best estimate for use in comparative effectiveness trials."[18]

If we want valid answers about the effectiveness of SMT we need to conduct valid studies and write valid systematic reviews with valid selection criteria and quality rating scales. We have failed on all accounts. You will be hard pressed to find more than a very few SMT studies that include a valid dose of thrust SMT care or systematic reviews that take these very significant variables into consideration.

We need to standardise how we study chiropractic SMT. We need to operationally define SMT as high-velocity low

---

16 Senna & Machaly (2011) Does Maintained Spinal Manipulation Therapy for Chronic Nonspecific Low Back Pain Result in Better Long-Term Outcome? SPINE 36 (18) 1427-37
17 Fritz, J.M. et al. (2015) Early physical therapy vs usual care in patients with recent-onset low back pain: A randomized clinical trial. JAMA 314 (14): 1459-1467
18 Haas, M. et al. (2014) Dose-Response and Efficacy of Spinal Manipulation for Care of Chronic Low Back Pain: A Randomized Controlled Trial Spine J. 2014 July 1; 14(7): 1106–1116

amplitude thrust SMT or chiropractic adjustment and not allow mobilisations to be defined as SMT/adjustments. Mobilisations need to be defined and studied as a separate intervention. We also need a standardised frequency of SMT treatments for a standardised duration. My suggestion would be to make research mimic clinical practice and the conclusions of the Haas et al. study. Why not set a standardised frequency of 3 times a week for 4 weeks, measure outcomes, then, if improvement is shown but not complete, do another period of 3 times a week for 2 weeks and then remeasure the outcomes.

This would provide a lot of data regarding whether or not, and how much, patients improve in terms of pain and function, or whatever other outcomes one wants to measure, at 4 weeks, and, if they are not completely resolved, if a further 2 weeks of care elicits further improvement. If more improvement has been seen and yet the patients are not fully resolved, then it would be easy to add another 2 weeks of care on an ongoing basis until symptoms are resolved and function is restored.

Further, it would make perfect sense to study the effects of ongoing chiropractic care over longer periods of time. If chiropractic care improves symptoms and functional ability by restoring spinal function, and if the industrial lifestyle causes spinal dysfunction, it makes perfect sense to study whether or not regular chiropractic care can maintain spinal function and/or improved spine-related health and/or overall health and wellbeing outcomes. The landmark study by Senna and Machaly published in Spine, showing significant benefit from maintenance SMT care vs no maintenance SMT care is ample justification for further study.

With properly controlled studies with a placebo or sham

manipulation group this would provide very important data. Any comparators should be for the same duration. If we are going to compare chiropractic SMT to drugs or any other comparator, then the dose of care and timing of outcomes data collection must be standardised and made equal between the groups.

It would not be difficult to standardise frequency and duration of care for studies, and to make mandatory inclusion of a control or sham SMT group and standardised duration of any comparators. This is research methodology 101; I cannot understand why we have not done this. Every systematic review on SMT laments that few published studies meet selection criteria with respect to methodological validity, yet we keep funding and conducting low quality studies! This is a waste of valuable limited resources and leads to more heterogeneity of results which leads to invalid downgrading of the level of evidence for SMT.

There is so much more to discuss but space will not allow. Instead, I will conclude with a plea for the standardisation of chiropractic SMT/adjustment studies with respect to dose of care, timing of data collection, and thrust SMT/adjustment vs non-thrust mobilisations and, in the meantime, for systematic reviews to address these issues of validity in their selection criteria, data analysis, and conclusions.

It is clinically and scientifically absurd to continue to conduct and/or pool together in systematic reviews, data from studies that have, "The number of SMT treatments varied from 1 to 24 and follow-up from immediate posttreatment to 3 years", or that include mobilisations instead of thrust manipulations but are classified as SMT studies.[12]

Stuart Kelly BSc, MSc(Chiro), DC

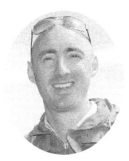

An AECC graduate and qualified life coach, Stuart runs 2 successful practices in Ireland along with his sister. He's had the privilege of adjusting international sports stars and world-renowned music artists and has appeared on TV and many radio shows discussing the benefits of Chiropractic.

For 4 years he organised international chiropractic speakers to present at the Ireland Chiropractic Association. Stuart's passion is helping people to be the best they can be and he works with other chiropractors to reconnect with their authenticity.

What do you believe?

"Are you sure?"

"Would it not be best to..."

"You'd never forgive yourself if..."

"What if this happens?"

If you're a vitalistic chiropractor you've probably heard these questions many times from people close to you, when it comes to family health decisions. When your partner, family or friends have a different belief system to you about health, sticking to your chiropractic principles can be challenging, especially if you have doubts around the body's ability to heal when the nervous system is functioning optimally. We live in a society where people want things fast and where quick fixes are the norm. Even when it comes to health challenges, popping pills or electing for surgery can often seem the easier option. Rather than functionally correcting the cause of the problem, many choose to block the symptoms. One of the biggest stumbling blocks for vitalistic chiropractors is the belief that they may not be delivering what they promise. So how do we build certainty in the chiropractic principles?

Examining belief systems

We all develop our belief systems through influential events and people we encounter from childhood, be it from our mother, father, teacher or preacher. I know when I was growing up the local medical doctor's word was gospel and not to be questioned. Thankfully this is changing a lot and people are asking more questions of the established professions and challenging them for alternatives to health problems. We only have to look at health on a global scale to see that we need a different approach. And that's where chiropractic is beautifully placed to lead a new and innovative approach in healthcare, focusing on the body's innate ability to heal. We know that a healthy diet, being emotionally stable and maintaining a fit and strong body will decrease chances of ill health. Combine this with regular chiropractic care, which maximises nervous system function – the master control system – and we see a person express and maximise their full potential.

How my experience shaped my beliefs

You know the benefits of Chiropractic but there's a difference between knowing on a pedagogic level and truly believing in the chiropractic principles. I feel we need to have an experience to convince us, to strengthen our conviction in the power of the adjustment. This can come in different forms. For some, it's a wealth of clinical experience with patients over many years. For me, it was my son's development under chiropractic care after undergoing a traumatic birth.

My wife Jacqueline was well adjusted all the way through her pregnancy. She studied her hypnobirthing and had even picked out her outfit for the home pool birth we were planning. As usual, the universe had other ideas. Her waters broke early, she was induced and this led to a cascade of interventions, resulting in an extremely traumatic birth for her and our son Fionn. Although we were full of gratitude to be able to hold our son in our arms, the inevitable trauma from such a birth resulted in a failure to thrive, difficulty feeding and delayed motor development.

The first 2 years of Fionn's life were challenging, with recurrent chest and ear infections and difficulty with head control, which resulted in delayed crawling and walking. I have looked after so many children in practice over the years, but when it's your own child you are more emotionally attached and the stakes are higher. It will also test your resolve, conviction and belief in how Chiropractic can influence and impact a developing nervous system.

Thankfully my wife also lives the chiropractic lifestyle and we both knew that no matter what challenges he was going through, an optimally functioning nervous system would only help his cause.

I'm pleased to say Fionn is now thriving. He's a fit and healthy boy, excelling at school and sport with vigour and confidence. The reconnection of his nervous system through chiropractic care was vital to his development. Looking back, I am grateful for his birth as it presented a challenge through which I had to grow and learn. It installed a degree of certainty in the effectiveness and power of Chiropractic. And so, my question to you is this; what cases in your practice strengthen your belief? Go and look for them. I can assure you they are there. What are you measuring objectively in practice? HRV, pulse oximetry, posture, BP and functional neurological changes are just a few things we can measure to assess the body's physiological change when under chiropractic care. There are most likely miracles happening every day in your practice, but are you asking the right questions or measuring the right things to notice them?

It's here I should stress that while Chiropractic is undoubtedly an immensely powerful tool, I have found it works best as part of an integrated approach. Too often I hear "gurus" on stage claiming it's a silver bullet to fix all ills. That's why I feel it's vital the modern chiropractor has awareness around the need for proper nutrition, being physically strong and robust, and having adequate stress management tools in today's healthcare arena.

The reflection between person and practice

The second most profound realisation during 20 years of practice was the fact that my practice is a reflection of me and the person I am. No matter what I tried to implement to boost my practice, be it new systems, protocols, team training and procedures – all of which are extremely helpful in the right context – how successful I was going to be in practice was intrinsically linked to my values, beliefs and all the baggage I was carrying around. Most of the time I didn't even know it was there holding me back!

This brings me to the doubts I've heard over the years from chiropractors who have asked themselves: "Am I in the right profession? How did my practice end up here? Is this where I want to be? Has Chiropractic just become a job? Do I still feel inspired to get up every morning and serve?" Every chiropractor, if they are honest, will have thought about one or more of these questions at some time in their career. I believe success in practice will come down to one major factor: realising the connection between you and your values, as these represent the very core of who you are.

Without knowing yourself in your truest form and having full acceptance for who you are, authenticity will allude you and the cracks in the masks you wear to hide your true identity will be ever harder to cover. These contradictions can lead to destruction in both personal and professional life.

Over the last 20 years I've found the following 5 steps have helped me remove the masks so I can live a more focused, fulfilling and congruent life that ripples through my everyday practice.

1. Finding out who I truly was.

I had to discover my true self, not who I thought I should be, and then own it and embrace it. I discovered what my priorities are and what's most important to me. I started by looking at the things I thought about most, the things I naturally gravitated towards and that I was motivated to do easily. I thought about the courses I went on, the books I read, the podcasts I listened to, the people I enjoyed being around, the conversations I really tuned into and the topics I easily remembered. All of these were clues to what is important to me and what makes up the very essence of who I am. I started with the Values Determination Process on Dr. John DeMartini's website, drdemartini.com

2. Finding my biggest block.

Throughout life we develop perceptions of events and people that we encounter. Unbalanced perceptions can lead to feelings of guilt, shame and resentment. This can be very destructive and affect self-esteem, resulting in feelings of unworthiness. Sometimes we are unaware that these perceptions are there but they show up in all aspects of our life. They sit subconsciously and inhibit self-expression in its highest form. I tackled the events in my life that I felt shame and guilt towards. I worked on any resentments I had towards people and neutralised them. I came to the realisation that everything is *on the way in life, not in the way and that everything has served me.*

3. Taking responsibility and moving forward constructively.

I had to learn to accept my current situation and take full responsibility for it. It was up to me to create the life I want. Over my years in practice, I have observed that one of the main things holding people back was their reluctance to make peace with their past, this is often their biggest block. I'm sure there are plenty of things in your life that you perceive you've done or not done, said or not said, or maybe you perceive you've been on the receiving end of someone's bad choices. We are all human and just doing the best we can in every given moment. You've most likely done more good than bad in your life. What if your "mistakes" were not mistakes at all, but correction points to bring you back on track to your true self, and if they never happened you'd be moving further off course.

4. Addressing limiting beliefs.

What were the main beliefs I was carrying around with me that weren't serving me? Other people have huge influence over the beliefs we have about ourselves, the majority of which had no truth whatsoever when I dug deeper into them. I asked myself: "The last time I was about to take on a challenge or task and then hesitated, what was the thought that made me stop?" The answer was often, "I'm not good enough. I don't deserve it. I can't do it." What are your limiting beliefs? The way I overcame mine was to create new empowering beliefs based on facts, rather than other people's opinions.

5. Assessing what it is I truly want in life.

Analysing my fears and stepping into them as well as expanding my comfort zone was vital for me to grow and achieve the things I want in life. After all, sturdy ships were not meant to stay in the harbour forever.

While everything I've shared is very much my own story and not advice, it's likely your struggles are not unique to you. We're all dealing with the same issues, limitations and challenges in personal life as well as in practice. Rather than walking away from fear, I learnt that I had to step into it and hold true to my principles.

Wisdom #32

Bill Esteb

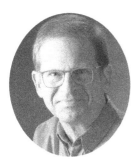

William has been a chiropractic patient and advocate since 1981. After working as the creative director for various advertising agencies in the USA, he helped write and produce Peter Grave's video for Renaissance International. He is the creative director of Patient Media and the cofounder of the Perfect Patients website service.

William is also the author of 12 books that explore the doctor–patient relationship from a patient's perspective, and his Monday Morning Motivation is emailed to over 10,000 subscribers each week.

33 Chiropractic Patient Principles

The most popular exhibit at the British Museum in London is the Rosetta Stone.

Inscribed on the stone are 3 versions of a decree issued by an Egyptian king in 196 BC. The 2 top blocks of text are different forms of Egyptian hieroglyphics, while the third is in Greek. The stone became the key to deciphering ancient Egyptian literature and civilisation.

Here are some principles for decoding patient behaviours, based on 40 years of experience as a chiropractic patient and advocate. Perhaps these will provide you with a key to understanding why patients do what they do, and what to do about it.

1. Patients buy the messenger before they buy the message. This simple truth is what Ralph Waldo Emerson was inferring when he observed, *"Who you are speaks so loudly I can't hear what you're saying."* This is about the law of identity and how you present yourself with patients. Posing, or assuming a persona, is based on the lie that if you showed up as yourself no one would like you. It's not true.

2. The most effective chiropractors are healthier than their patients. But not with a "healthier than thou" attitude. Patients rarely become healthier than their doctor. Keep this in mind if you wish to serve wellness-minded individuals. Most chiropractors are in great physical health. The opportunity is in the mental and social domains.

3. Power and influence come from authenticity. You'll want to avoid spending your limited social authority issuing "doctor's orders". What's more attractive is to come alongside and show up as an inspirer and cheerleader. This is especially helpful since the patients are doing the healing, not you. You're unleashing their doctor within.

4. The best communicators are profound listeners. Many have been misled into thinking a finely honed script or having all the answers is the key. No. It's the social skill of listening. Take care to avoid interrupting patients, making assumptions or jumping to conclusions. Listen for unusual word choices. Ask about those.

5. Talking too much. When speaking with patients, using words as a drug is an outside-in process. Speaking is among the least

effective communication channels, yet many chiropractors use words with abandon. After all, they're free. But like anything in great abundance, as quantity increases, value decreases.

6. Precise language creates better outcomes. How patients see the world occurs in language. Are you working with spinal dysfunction or subluxation? Manipulation or adjustment? Feeling or function? Sloppy language creates a sloppy life. A sloppy life creates a sloppy practice. Specificity is proof that you care.

7. Chiropractic is different. Making Chiropractic more like medicine to please patients or seek medical acceptance does neither. Medicine is interested in the problem in the person. Chiropractic is interested in the person with the problem. Big difference. A difference that makes all the difference in the world.

8. Chiropractic is about nerves, not bones. Ignoring the potential whole-body effects of nervous system interference, turns Chiropractic into orthopractic. And let's not forget that bones are static structures that only move when commanded by muscles. And muscles only contract when commanded by the nervous system.

9. Patients want an outcome but you deliver a process. Most patients think their problem is their pain. It's what motivates many to seek your care. Because of their allopathic notion of healthcare, they think your prescription of 3 visits a week is producing the outcome they want.

10. Avoid treating symptoms with adjustments. Whether you explicitly or implicitly agree to treat a patient's symptoms, you've left Chiropractic and entered medicine. Drugs are faster, cheaper and more convenient. This is probably the most common (and preventable) patient communication oversight. Ignore it and patients will most certainly discontinue their care when they feel better.

11. Subluxation is the body's creative attempt to accommodate stress. Subluxation is a brilliant short-term survival strategy. Granted, there are negative consequences from longstanding subluxations. This is why you'd want to find out if the physical, chemical or emotional stressor is still present.

12. There are actually 4 subluxations. This is why certain chronic subluxation patterns don't resolve. Subluxations can be from physical, intellectual, emotional or spiritual causes. If a patient is in a constant state of emotional turmoil, your physical intervention is likely to be palliative at best.

13. Germs trump subluxations. Most patients are more concerned about cooties on the headrest paper than subluxations. The recent experience with Covid-19 is a good example of this misplaced fear. Until you help patients put their germaphobia in perspective, Chiropractic is merely therapeutic.

14. Your purpose is not to adjust patients. I hope you adjust patients and you do it masterfully, delivering what BJ Palmer characterised as "the adjustment with that something extra". However, adjusting patients isn't your purpose. Rather it helps

advance, fulfil or accomplish your purpose. Do you know what yours is?

15. Adjusting more segments doesn't improve clinical outcomes. This is based on the lie that "more is more". It's not true. Adjusting secondary and tertiary subluxations or cavitating every articulation is often justified as being thorough. Often it covers a lack of confidence.

16. Patients aren't living to get adjusted. They get adjusted so they can live. Coming to your practice is an interruption and inconvenience. Which is why everything you say and do should conspire to make a patient's visit the highlight of their day.

17. Healing is a spiritual phenomenon. DD Palmer understood this when he observed that the purpose of Chiropractic is to *"connect man the physical with man the spiritual"*. Healing stops when the spirit vacates the body. Be sure to make the distinction between spirit, which animates the body, and man-made religion.

18. Patients cannot be educated into wanting wellness. There's nothing you can say or do to change how a patient prioritises their health. You can scare, shame or guilt patients, but it rarely lasts. The value each patient places on his or her health was formed long before meeting you. And a snappy report of findings is unlikely to change it.

19. Most patient education is merely patient teaching. If you're talking, you're teaching, which rhymes with preaching. And

this is usually what it is. Instead, ask questions. Show up curious and interested in what patients believe. It's more respectful and holds the promise of becoming a productive conversation.

20. Beliefs produce behaviours. Patients do what they do because they believe what they believe. All of us act in ways to remain congruent with our beliefs, even if we're not conscious of those beliefs. If you seek long-term patient relationships, you're actually in the belief-changing business.

21. It's unlikely that you're permanently fixing spines. By the time an adult shows up in your practice, they have the effects of a lifetime of neglect. They expect their spinal issue to resolve like an infection or indigestion. But it's more like a stain, producing a permanently weakened area, susceptible to relapse.

22. Few patients embrace Chiropractic as a lifestyle adjunct on their first exposure. The exception is chiropractors. Most chiropractors had a Eureka! moment and decided to become a chiropractor. Then, they spend the rest of their career attempting to recreate that same moment for patients. It doesn't work that way.

23. Create a safe place to fail. Many patients must start and stop Chiropractic care multiple times before they get the big idea, which means you'd want to make it easy for a patient to discontinue care without guilt or shame. Play the long game. Set the stage for their relapse and eventual reactivation.

24. How you say goodbye affects referrals and reactivations.

Patients know when it's their last visit. But they rarely announce it. They imagine your awkward attempt to talk them out of it. Thus, there isn't proper closure. They avoid you in the grocery store. And when their problem returns, they go elsewhere because they think you're angry with them.

25. Getting new patients is simple. Tell the chiropractic story to as many strangers as possible. If you're uncomfortable around strangers, or don't encounter many these days, your new patient numbers suffer. Referrals from great results aren't enough. Participate in clubs and service organisations. Become familiar by generously contributing.

26. Sell your talent, not your time. If you want to help as many people as possible, use your most valuable inventory wisely: your time. There's only so much of it. Make sure every patient understands that they're buying your talent, wisdom and experience - not face time.

27. To attract patients you must be willing to repel. Like a magnet, to attract you must polarise. Going beige, biting your tongue and walking on eggshells to avoid offending others is a recipe for being invisible. You're a rebel. Feral. Plant your flag. As Dr Gentempo correctly asserts, *"Your stand is your brand."*

28. More new patients will solve everything. True, an underperforming staff, inconsistent policies, clumsy procedures and poor patient communications are less obvious when new patients are waiting in the wings. Abundant new patients cover a multitude of practice sins.

29. You don't have a new patient problem. If you've been practicing a decade or longer and still have a constant need for new patients, you actually have a patient *keeping* problem. It's a very different problem arising from practicing pain relief rather than delivering healthcare.

30. The patient brings more to the table than what you do on the table. Their ability to self-heal is the real hero. Without minimising the adjustment, a patient's recovery actually reveals more about them than you. Thus, the adage, *"Take no credit, take no blame"*.

31. Your power as a chiropractor is rather limited. At its best, chiropractic is a partnership. You have a job and the patient has a job. Results come from what you do on each visit and what they do between visits. And while you can't make patients do their job, make sure they know what it is.

32. Good health is a means, not an end. Patients aren't seeking the Ms Perfect Spine award or the Mr Subluxation-free trophy. Health permits us to live life to the full. Why does each patient want his or her health back? Ask.

33. Your practice only grows as you grow. Improved procedures and other efficiencies only grow a practice incrementally. Outside-in tactics are temporary, with the practice returning to a set point based on who you are. Personal development is the only way to make a permanent, lasting practice improvement. Like healing, practice growth comes from the inside out.

I hope that provokes a different way of seeing the doctor/patient relationship. Perhaps it will provide some insights that inspire success beyond your wildest dreams. Either way, let me know.

Melissa Sandford

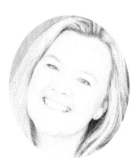

Melissa has been an integral part of Chiropractic in Europe for over 30 years. Owning and managing 3 independent practices has taught her the value of entrepreneurship blended with an incredible business savvy. As well as working individually with people, Melissa has created world-class seminars and front-desk training programmes in a trusting environment.

Currently serving as CEO, Melissa has played an integral part in the growth of the United Chiropractic Association. A speaker, teacher, gin-lover and mother of 6, she is a champion for all things chiropractic and living Life from the Inside Out.

Experiencing "that moment"

It's been 30 years since my first chiropractic adjustment and as I think back over that time, I often wonder how different my life would be without it. You see, I really did fall into Chiropractic; I married a chiropractor. And while it was never my intention to work in Chiropractic, here I am 30 years later with 27 years' service and wearing many different chiropractic hats.

Chiropractic has given me more than just great health; it has given me the principles with which I choose to live my life. Without those principles where would I be living? What work would I be doing? Would I have 6 children? What kind of medication would I be taking? The list goes on.

What I do know is that I have a certainty and belief in Chiropractic that guides me in everything I do. For me, living my life by chiropractic principles is just so simple and yet I live in a world watching others struggle with not only their health but their beliefs around health. I see a sense of powerlessness around life and an inability to make choices and decisions. I see people and communities not able to trust the innate wisdom of their bodies. Instead, they are fearful and often make health decisions from that place.

One question I often ask myself is, "Why doesn't everyone get it, how can they not see that life can be done differently?"

I have a distinct memory of the moment, yes that moment; the one when you "get it", when you really understand Chiropractic.

That moment when you know that we are self-healing, self-regulating organisms.

That moment when you know that your body has an inborn intelligence and we need to learn to tune-in to it.

That moment when you know that healing takes time.

That moment when you know we are connected above down and inside out.

My moment wasn't via my husband's teachings, nor his report of findings or even the fact that I had dramatic changes to my health. No, it was a moment in time when I was ready. I had spent time healing, learning and most of all questioning everything I knew and understood about health.

There I was at a chiropractic conference and it hit me like

a bolt of lightning. I had been listening to the same stories, the same information that I had heard many times before but this time it was different. Chiropractic moved from being a treatment for ailments to a way of life.

I am grateful for that moment; it has given me a life I could never have dreamed of. Not only have I had the great privilege of helping many people to discover the benefits of Chiropractic in my varied roles, I have also had the great privilege of raising 6 beautiful chiropractic children. All born at home with no intervention, no vaccinations and only a handful of A&E visits. Being part of their journey to discovering their own views on health and the principles with which they "do life" has been and still is, my greatest joy.

My wish for Chiropractic is that chiropractors gently lead their patients and communities to arrive at "that moment". That they don't just rely on that awesome pre-care class or report of findings. That they give them time and as Bill Esteb says, "*allow them the space to fail*".

My wish for our future world is a life lived without fear, a life where we trust in the innate healing ability of the body. A life where people have tools to make decisions and choices aligned with their values and beliefs. Chiropractic has given me all of these things in abundance and I will always be truly grateful for "that moment".

Wisdom #33

Brandi MacDonald

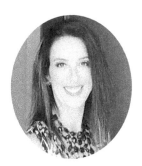

Brandi is a Chiropractic advocate, speaker, author and visionary who runs a busy Chiropractic practice in Edmonton, Alberta with her husband Dr Don MacDonald. Together they also run True Concepts Chiropractic Seminars delivering seminars globally.

As a couple they have built a world-wide tribal following called "The Vitality Shift" helping Chiropractors and practices to find their premise and align it to increase their personal and professional success. Brandi is a board member of the Australian Spinal Research foundation has spoken on all of the biggest stages within Chiropractic around the world.

Wisdom in the musings of a life in Chiropractic

For 13 years, along with my husband Don, I've helped to drive our practice in Edmonton, Alberta. And to drive progress, by travelling the world, speaking on chiropractic stages and mentoring our tribe through The Vitality Shift. After a career supporting vulnerable woman and children, I found my niche in helping chiropractic principles and offices around the world to understand their purpose and to develop their potential. My daily Facebook posts were serialised in a book called *Sipping Brandi* and here are 3 extracts of wisdom that I hope stimulate your mind:

"I have noticed that it seems easier for the world to love a suffering woman than it is to love a confident, joyful one." – Glennan Doyle

As much as we fear failure, we can also fear success. Some of the deepest work we have done is to recognise how much reinforcement we get from being dramatic, overwhelmed, struggling, sad, broke, sick, or any state less than. Imagine then if you took ALL your support away. Would you feel mighty?

When our definition of who we are is tied up in drama or disease, it's incredibly challenging to sort out who we might be without that definition, because the by-product is that we will lose many people who unknowingly think they help us by being our support. We have seen this so often in how many people ask us, "How can people like the way you talk to them?" or "Don't people get offended?" Because I am not a comfort bond for clients or my friends. Over time I have learned where to give my version of support and where to take it away. And that has led to me becoming a ninja transformer, not because people love me or want to hear the dirty truth, but because I won't support dysfunction. I only want the best for people. I understand struggle but will not bow to it as my slave to help others.

Rather I choose to bow to potential, and desire. Someone must have both, in order to transform, for people with great potential but zero desire tend to stay in struggle and get standing ovations for it. I don't work with these folks. However, anyone with desire and bravery, who understands that they will in fact lose much support as they gain their freedom to be authentic, I will do whatever it takes for them. It has created a black-and-white life for me. I clearly know I am not a popularity queen, but my work has transcended that need. I desire transformation, not acceptance. And those who desire that with me often have life-changing experiences. Struggle reinforcement? Or authenticity. Every day we get to choose. No one said it was easy but trust me it is possible.

"If you don't know who you truly are, you'll never know what you really want."

What makes a "successful" entrepreneur? Collections? Volume? Profitability? Number of staff? Number of locations? Ever met an unhappy successful person? The answer is emphatically "yes". So, are hard business numbers the only gauge of success? We started a mastermind programme called The Shift Rewire Masterclass, because business acumen is important. Sales and profit do matter unless you run a free service. But success is so much more complex. It is not as black-and-white and relative. What one person may consider to be success, another may not. However, I think successful entrepreneurs (however they define it) come with common denominators by our observations and our own learning.

They understand their core values and live in alignment with them, despite pressure to do otherwise.

Business acumen is just that. A skill. Not an emotional charge on money, sales, profit, investing or saving. When a skill is lacking, they learn it, they don't avoid it, because there isn't an emotion attached to it.

They understand hustle and rest, and don't get the two confused. Business takes hustle; it takes grit, grind, boring repetition - and they do it. And then they rest. Burnout is not an option.

They spend more time on the WHO than the WHAT... with an uber awareness that business comes through them, not to them.

They care for their vehicle as much as they care for their business - this is their physical body and without it, it's hard to do the above. They read voraciously but apply the 80% production over 20% consumption. "Busy" means GSD, not the mind busy taking in irrelevant information

Focus is their superpower. Being selfish, guilty, anxiety, anger, etc plays no role in their choices; see the first bullet point as to why.

They are crystal clear about why they are on this planet and will do whatever it takes to achieve that end goal.

Perhaps we should start putting a word in front of success and call it "aligned success". Alignment of self with everything we choose means nothing if it ever feels like a loss or mistake. Rather we should look to whether we are aligned or out of alignment and then reset accordingly. When we seek that, success follows.

"We are the answer..."

Yesterday was like any other day at our practice South Side Chiropractic. Except that it wasn't. It was more vivid than some days where we are running around like headless chickens. It started with a 13-year-old who had previously spent two years of his short life in the medical system, waking his parents every night for 2 years because he needed a hot bath to ease his stomach pain, missing on average 66 days of school because of mysterious digestive pain. This poor kid had been scoped, needled, drugged and had drunk toxic chemicals for scans with still no answer. Until his medical doctor referred him to us. Yesterday we wrote "no stomach pain" on his re-evaluation and graduated his care down.

There was a woman who had ulcerative colitis, who's been off work for 6 months bleeding and in excruciating pain, healed by her 8th visit and goes back to work next week. Then a new patient 30 years old, who had not pooped daily since high school, has now pooped every day since her first adjustment with us. She was shocked. Also, a young man born with club foot, who could not coordinate his body; he can balance now and after his adjustment was going golfing for the first time since high school.

Then there was our little neuro-affected child who had massive meltdowns and we saw her during Covid-19. She has had the best few weeks after the last few adjustments. At one of our re-evaluations, a practice member had gained 2 inches of height in less than 6 weeks because his head position returned to normal. You know what they all have in common? Chiropractic. You know what else they did in conjunction with chiropractic? Nothing.

Our day like any other day, also had a myriad of stories of healing and stories of people who are simply staying well, who can also no longer remember what it felt like to be unwell. In a matter of minutes, what a chiropractic adjustment does alone, is something we do not honour enough. Our office is not unique. It is the same as hundreds, maybe thousands across the world. Yet so few know and so many more feel something else is needed. It is not. We have the power in our hands. And in our clinical skills. And in our communication. Use that. Up-level that. Because the more of us who see the simplicity and power of a couple minutes of time, and hands that create ease in a distressed system, maybe we will have the chance to change the world with our uniqueness and two hands alone.

We are the answer.

Rose Milward MSc, DC

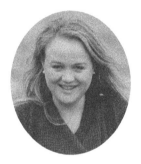

Rose Millward DC is a passionate and confident Chiropractor, who manages a busy pair of practices in the Scottish Borders. A 2016 graduate from the Welsh Institute of Chiropractic, she has been a sought-after Associate and has thrived as a Chiropractor.

In 2019 she moved to Scotland to work with her colleague and mentor Donald Francis DC, firstly as a chiropractor, then as Practice Manager. In a year she has built a successful practice and transformed the clinic systems. Originally from London, Rose prides herself on being committed, consistent and relaxed in practice, believing the key to success rests on one's ability to be authentic.

My Gift to Chiropractic

If you can truly master the profound ability to be a chiropractor as well as yourself, it is my honest belief that you will have the potential to infinitely grow and be content in all situations; knowing you have complete strength and authenticity.

My highest goal is to have the feeling of calm and happiness in my daily life. I have identified this sense of wellbeing as my highest value, as losing it took all enjoyment out of my life. So, in the past 2 years I have endeavoured to learn how to opt into a life which is free of anxiety and distress. I have discovered the key to my sense of happiness and calm, as well as identifying what causes me to lose my way in the first place.

I have found, through extensive study of myself, that when attempting to be someone I am not, I feel the most amount of distress and exhaustion. Besides the anxiety that trying to embody a false identity causes us all, the perpetual sense of incongruity takes a lot of energy to maintain and ultimately will lead to a sense of unhappiness and fatigue.

I have found that most of us will have a safety mechanism, like a safety hook in a rockface, which stops us from plummeting into emotional blackholes. My biggest hook, the one that keeps me safe, is having complete authenticity. Whether I am having to make a life decision, like where to live or who to work for, or what professional advice I should give, channelling all actions through the filter of "What do I really want?" or "What do I really believe?" provides the sure footing I need to keep me safe on any of life's rock faces.

To put this into context so you can relate it to your life, we need to start with the reality.

Our profession is currently misunderstood by most, we work with natural healing (which is unpredictable at the best of times), and unfortunately, we have often been put in the same box as GPs or physiotherapists. On top of this, we need to deal with conflicting professional philosophies and a lot of voices, all telling us what we should and shouldn't believe. Many of us chiropractors can relate to a sense of feeling that we should be more than we are, that we should have a biblical ability to heal others, that we should somehow understand all the infinite changes a body can make, and that everybody we come across will like and understand us if only we just said the right thing and delivered the goods.

If any of these thoughts feel familiar to you, or others which you may have adopted or absorbed in your professional or personal life, I would say take a closer look. And if you can't logically figure out what you know to be true, then I would recommend you trust the visceral reaction in your stomach as to whether you are on board with something or not. When we have beliefs which contradict or misguide us, we will feel that guttural sense of unease. This unease can manifest itself in many forms; as anxiety before work, looking at the diary with gloom, dreading seeing certain people, negative self-talk, or anything in our week which steals our sense of happiness and calm.

My way of navigating both professional and life challenges revolves around the premise that I must be authentic with myself and everyone, at all times. Unless you work to fully understand what that means to you, you will be stifled in your professional and personal growth and fulfilment.

Professional growth for chiropractors comes in the form of delivering repeatable, reliable care for people and being happy and calm through the process. How well we do professionally and personally, I think, matches our ability to be authentic in practice. It takes energy to see as many people as we would like to without feeling exhausted or burnt out. Feeling strong, calm and confident with any person going through any form of struggle, requires us to be completely grounded and authentic in ourselves, with no confusion at our core about what we are doing and why.

Being a chiropractor, or any health professional, requires a high efficiency of intention to action energy transfer. Like an athlete throwing a shotput, or a karate master breaking a concrete block. When we are working in practice, we cannot be losing energy in second guessing our own beliefs, acting incongruently and generally being inauthentic.

Whether it is through adapting or changing our communication, the adjustment we deliver, the questions we ask or the energy we meet people with; it is my truth that this is all best guided by our own intuition. That intuition which can only be heard when we are being truly honest ourselves. Something which I do when communicating with patients who are struggling with either the understanding of their problem or the care process, is to think, "How would I explain this to someone I love, like my mother", as this will best place me to be how I am with the people I love, where I am truly myself. From this place I can express compassion, explanation and guidance without ego, uncertainty or incongruency.

Chiropractors describe "getting into state" or "flow", which I understand to some more analytical personalities or inexperienced professionals could sound a bit loopy. To me, this is when a chiropractor can empty their mind of all distractions and they are just guided by their intuition. Intuition which of course is also fed information by our innate (for example the physical muscle memory of how to adjust, the breathing we create, the muscle tone we recruit) and by our intellectual mind (which has learnt the science and systems behind our care) as well as our true honest authentic self. The primary reason for not being connected, not being able to access our intuition, or our own innate, I think, is that we are trying to be someone we are not.

The common areas where I think we, as a profession and a society, buckle in this department is in fact trying to embody others. Whether this is trying to be a "crusader chiropractor" perhaps practicing in a way which we do not want or we do not feel competent enough to do, maybe recommending different frequencies of care to the paying public than we would for our own mother, or even dressing or speaking in a way which is unrecognisable by our own sense of self. Fully disguising who we are, and how we feel, and how we think, is unwise in all cases and will destroy any sense of happiness, calm, or contentment.

And if, through some unfortunate circumstance you uncover your own self and you cannot accept or are not fond of some elements, then, as I say to all the people I see, the first step to healing is awareness. As awareness leads to action. It is better to take action towards helping yourself, rather than choosing to ignore, conceal and live a life with inauthenticity and self-belief foundations made of figurative sand.

So, my gift you; be only yourself in the room with the people you are seeing, do not conceal your natural form or, like me, your outer London-high-energy honest personality. By accepting who you are, you can be guided by your own intuition, channel all of your energy into what you are doing and not into hiding who you are. Accept yourself so that others can accept you, and then you can lovingly and easily care for people, and in doing so care for yourself and for your family.

Eulogy

My son, David Russell was born in Brisbane on the 8th May 1975. Throughout his life David was kind, caring, and forever willing to go the extra mile for whatever he believed in. From infancy he spent time daily with his namesake and grandfather, David Bassingthwaighte who was an unusually courageous and caring soul. It was from him David learned to listen to views of others, and that if you feel strongly about what you believe, to ignore the criticism and continue working towards your goal. My father successfully lived by this ethic.

At Brisbane Boys College, David always volunteered for fundraising with his friend. The highly successful duo would go off together after school, collecting funds for whatever cause the school was supporting. David always won the prize for fundraising.

David was voted cross country captain, not because he was the best runner, but because of his commitment to the team and its younger members. There was opposition to this appointment from the cross-country master, who asked him to withdraw his nomination because he felt David couldn't run in the top Greater Public Schools 6. Parents rallied, and he remained joint captain. After having a chiropractic adjustment just prior to the GPS event, he ran 5th, with a personal best time. Despite being asked what drugs he was on, he recognised his successful performance was the result of the chiropractic adjustment, and was hooked. From this time and under the influence of his chiropractor and mentor, Michael Troy, he valued chiropractic and his enthusiasm and love for it never dwindled.

David enrolled at the New Zealand College of Chiropractic in its early days. He rallied support for the college when it looked as though government funding might be withdrawn, by asking his boss, where he was working as a telemarketer, if he could use the phone and call chiropractors around the world to enlist their support. During his student years he formed wonderful friendships, worked moderately well, organised a huge number of memorable parties, and quite simply had the time of his life.

After a few years working in Melbourne, he returned to Auckland where he became the Chiropractic Centre Director of the New Zealand Chiropractic College. David embraced the challenges associated with this position with great enthusiasm and he held the position for 8 years. He was determined to maintain the highest of standards, taking every opportunity to encourage support for the college throughout the world. It continues to be recognised and spoken of today.

David had a great dedication to, and love of, teaching. With his larger-than-life personality and infectious laugh, he made learning fun and as interesting as possible. He encouraged the younger chiropractors of the future. Concurrently, he held an expectation that his students be focused and have a solid commitment.

David was father of 3 wonderful children, Saskia, Oliver and Zara, a simply amazing dad who never lost his inner child; dressing up with the children for Halloween, leaving evidence of Santa and the Easter Bunny, and no doubt enjoying such activities as much or even more than the children. He was always available to take part in everything that held their interest, and I'm sure they will retain those great memories forever. He had love and respect for his extended family and was always there to help and assist. Nothing was too much trouble, even when the going was tough.

Even as a child, he loved to cook, picking up the latest gourmet magazine, giving me a list of ingredients that he required. We would all share in the results. In Auckland, he built a pizza oven, bought a smoker, and produced some of the best food ever. He had a great love of gardening and developed a garden with such wonderful energy - lots of fruit trees, grape vines, a small plot of vegetables - all beautifully tended.

David was also a member of, and held executive positions in, the Alumni Association, NZCA, Hamelin Trust, and the Australian Spinal Research Foundation. His drive and interest in contributing to expanding knowledge in the profession was second to none. He authored and co-authored 37 research papers. He was ever focused on being inclusive, fostering respect, tolerance and sharing between and among those within the profession. His awards included NZCCAA Chiropractor of the Year 2005, NZCCAA Outstanding Service Award 2007, NZCC Outstanding Service Award 2011, NZCA Service Award 2012 and 2016.

In 2015, David became a founding member and Vice-Chairman of the Scotland College of Chiropractic Charitable Trust. He talked with such joy and enthusiasm of the progression of the college. We often joked about his SCCCT art installation of papers pinned to his living room wall. I have no doubt that his tireless effort, practical experience, and research knowledge contributed to the strong foundations that will be the Edinburgh college. And I believe he would have contributed much more as first principal.

David said, and it has been stated before by others, *"Chiropractic is beautiful! The bigger picture things that I'm involved with are to ensure the longevity of the profession and the principles of the profession, respect within that profession and choice for humanity."*

Jan Russell

Lightning Source UK Ltd.
Milton Keynes UK
UKHW020735070721
386770UK00006B/547